"Pranam to Robin Rothenberg for this remarkable book! *Svadhyaya Breath Journ*
text based on Robin's many years of research, practice and teaching, but a wo
companion for anyone sincere about restoring their prana and optimizing their h

—Leigh Blashki, Board of Directors, IAYT, C-IAYT,
and past-President Yoga Australia

"Rothenberg is taking the ancient art of pranayama and teaching it in a modern context. This journal is essential for all yoga teachers, yoga therapists and even students of yoga to use as they begin to explore the potency of their own breath patterns. Many people will be very surprised when they dig deep into the exercises that are elegantly laid out in this journal. They will find the life force within and learn how to use breath as a tool to self-regulate."

—Amy Wheeler, Ph.D., Board President of the
International Association of Yoga Therapists (2018–2020)

"Rothenberg has created the Sakti activator to her Siva volume *Restoring Prana*. This detailed companion workbook/journal brings each and every concept in *Restoring Prana* to life through specific, pragmatic, and progressive practices and questions for reflection that support the reader's experiential understanding of functional breathing, functional movement, and pranayama practices that support body/mind/spirit health. As she does so deftly in *Restoring Prana*, Robin masterfully braids the Western science around the respiratory function's crucial role in balanced body/mind/spirit health with the ancient teachings of Yoga and Ayurveda. Whether in a training program, continuing education, or individual personal exploration, this brilliant gem is an essential experiential guide for yoga practitioners, yoga teachers and therapists, and healthcare practitioners."

—Aggie Stewart, MA, C-IAYT, Yoga Teacher/Yoga Therapist,
former Accreditation Manager at IAYT, and author of Yoga as Self-Care for Healthcare
Practitioners: Cultivating Resilience, Compassion, and Empathy

"The SBJ workbook is an accessible and effective self-study tool for any yoga teacher, yoga therapist, or health care practitioner who is interested in learning and increasing their own mastery over breathing. Robin nicely bridges what we in Western medicine know about breathing and what yoga teaches to give the reader access to their Energetic Bank Account with the goal to bring healing to ourselves and others."

—Claudia Kleffner, OT, C-IAYT, Therapeutic Yoga Teacher and Yoga
Therapist, Faculty of Essential Yoga Therapy Training Program

"This amazing workbook is for people who don't just want to study yogic philosophy as a system of abstract concepts, but rather wish to incorporate the teachings of yoga into their everyday lives. Robin provides a step-by-step guide for cultivating health that interweaves the philosophic wisdom of the ancients with the most current understanding of human physiology and how the body functions."

—Lynn Crimando, C-IAYT, NBC-HWC, Buteyko Affiliated Practitioner

"A perfect companion to Robin Rothenberg's *Restoring Prana*. This manual guides the reader step by step in transformation of intellectual information contained in *Restoring Prana* into experiential embodied wisdom. The book covers short explanations followed by many practices using asanas, mantras, mudras, chanting, and breathing techniques. The guide focuses always on developing an understanding of our inner world and subtle body as we build awareness through recommended practices. It teaches breath/prana impact on every part of the body, emotions, and mind through specific practice sequences. It is open-ended rather than prescriptive as it invites and guides one through experimentation and inner awareness. As we follow *Svadhyaya Breath Journal* it will make us a better yoga teacher, yoga therapist and human being."

—Lee Majewski, MA, DYEd, C-IAYT, author and Yoga Therapist

by the same author

Restoring Prāṇa
A Therapeutic Guide to Prāṇāyāma and Healing Through the Breath for Yoga Therapists, Yoga Teachers, and Healthcare Practitioners
Robin L. Rothenberg
Foreword by Richard Miller
Illustrated by Kirsteen Wright
ISBN 978 1 84819 401 4
eISBN 978 0 85701 357 6

of related interest

Yoga Student Handbook
Develop Your Knowledge of Yoga Principles and Practice
Edited by Sian O'Neill
Foreword by Lizzie Lasater
ISBN 978 0 85701 386 6
eISBN 978 0 85701 388 0

Yoga Teaching Handbook
A Practical Guide for Yoga Teachers and Trainees
Edited by Sian O'Neill
ISBN 978 1 84819 355 0
eISBN 978 0 85701 313 2

Yoga Therapy as a Creative Response to Pain
Matthew J. Taylor
Foreword by John Kepner
ISBN 978 1 84819 356 7
eISBN 978 0 85701 315 6

Svādhyāya Breath Journal

A Companion Workbook to *Restoring Prāṇa*

ROBIN L. ROTHENBERG

Illustrated by Kirsteen Wright

SINGING DRAGON
LONDON AND PHILADELPHIA

First published in 2020
by Singing Dragon
an imprint of Jessica Kingsley Publishers
73 Collier Street
London N1 9BE, UK
and
400 Market Street, Suite 400
Philadelphia, PA 19106, USA

www.singingdragon.com

Library of Congress Cataloging in Publication Data
A CIP catalog record for this book is available from the Library of Congress

British Library Cataloguing in Publication Data
A CIP catalogue record for this book is available from the British Library

ISBN 978 1 78775 258 0

Printed and bound in Great Britain

Contents

Introduction 7

1. The Breath as a Window into Your World. 11
Practice 1.1: Daily Accounting 13
Practice 1.2: The Breath and the Guṇas 18
Practice 1.3: The Breath and the Kleśas 20
Practice 1.4: Your Breath in Āsana 21
Practice 1.5: Saṃskāra Transformation 22
Practice 1.6: Breath in Āsana and Prāṇāyāma Practice—Changing our Sādhanā Practice 23
Practice 1.7: Remembering the Divine—Mantra and the Breath 25
Practice 1.8: Mantra and Breath in Action 26

2. The Five Winds and Your Energy Bank Account. 27
Practice 2.1: Assessing Your EBA 32
Practice 2.2: Your EBA Close Up and Personal 33
Practice 2.3: The Obstacles to Practice 35
Practice 2.4: Kriya Yoga through the Vayus 37

3. Breathing Basics: Respiration 101 39
Practice 3.1: Measuring your CO_2 45
Practice 3.2: The Breath Log 47

4. Subtle Breathing, the Foundation of Function 53
Practice 4.1: Subtle Breathing 56
Practice 4.2: Subtle Breathing—Full Practice 57

5. The Nose versus the Mouth 67
Practice 5.1: Nose Clearing (Photos 5 and 6) 70
Practice 5.2: Series to Develop the Tongue 71
Practice 5.3: Developing Healthy Speech 79
Practice 5.4: Mouth Taping at Night (Photos 14 and 15) 82

6. **The Diaphragm, the Breath, and the Core** **85**
Practice 6.1: Undulation Series 93
Practice 6.2: Core Breathing Series 98
Practice 6.3: Developing the Diaphragm Series 103

7. **The Core, the Bandhas, and the Breath** **109**
Practice 7.1: Developing Your Transverse Abdominis Series 114
Practice 7.2: Developing Your Pelvic Floor Series 126
Practice 7.3: Developing the Mid-Back Core Series 133
Practice 7.4: Developing the Neck Core Series 140

8. **The Emotional Brain and the Breath** **151**
Practice 8.1: Sensory Svādhyāya Practice 154
Practice 8.2: Wiring up the Vagus Series—Breath Practices to Transform the Mind 163

9. **The Mind of the Subtle Body** **173**
Practice 9.1: Svādhyāya on the Chakras 178
Practice 9.2: Coloring **Our Senses** **179**
Practice 9.3: Chakra Bija Mantra Practice 182
Practice 9.4: Mūdra and the Nādis (Photos 103–104) 183
Practice 9.5: Combining Mantra, Mūdra, Prāṇāyāma, and Āsana 187
Practice 9.6: Hand Mūdra for Nostril Techniques (Photos 105 and 106) 191

10. **Prāṇāyāma as Kumbhāka** **199**
Practice 10.1: Developing Suspension 202
Practice 10.2: Suspension with Movement Series—Breathe Less, Move More! 204

Glossary **217**
Endnotes **221**

INTRODUCTION

A Companion Workbook for Restoring Prāṇa Practices

The intention of this workbook is to offer you a ready-made Svādhyāya Breath Journal (SBJ) to track your experience of the practices relayed in *Restoring Prāṇa: A Therapeutic Guide to Prāṇāyāma and Healing Through the Breath*. The word "svādhyāya" translates as "self-reflection." A great deal of self-awareness is required in order to change breathing patterns due to our inherently deep-seated habituation to them. As we learn to control and manipulate the breath—and through that our prāṇa—it is helpful to journal or track the subtle and more revelatory changes that we experience. This enlivens the whole change process and lends perspective from the long view over time.

One of the dramatic discoveries I made in my own breath-retraining process was that literally everything I ate, thought, did, and felt impacted my breathing. Furthermore, the way in which I breathed while eating, thinking, doing, and feeling impacted the experience I was having. Definitive patterns emerged as I learned to view my life less as random, isolated events, and rather began to link them through the fluctuations of my breath. For instance, I noticed how hard and fast I breathed while arguing with my husband. The more heated our discussions, the more I felt like a dragon-lady spewing fire-bombs of words fueled by a lot of hot air. As I learned to quiet my breath, it actually changed the tenor of my side of the conversation. Essentially, it cooled down my thoughts, allowing me time to respond more thoughtfully to my spouse.

This experience of observing my life through the lens of the breath reminded me of how it felt to learn the secret of seeing the pictures camouflaged behind the dots of Magic Eye 3D images. To see the hidden image requires a systematic relaxation of the optic nerve. It's only when all striving is pacified that the picture suddenly pops into view. If you squint or try to force the reveal, the dots just seem to become more chaotic. In a similar way, I had to train myself to release assumption and judgment, to relax into my breath, and not force the process in order for the patterns to emerge. Journaling enabled me to track my experience, and over the ensuing weeks and months of retraining, helped me to understand myself in ways that had previously been hidden. The SBJ follows a similar mode. With it in hand, you as the practitioner have a means of linking your experience of each chapter's practices over time. This will assist you in discovering your underlying patterns, allowing them to "pop" and become more conscious to you.

Yoga requires action. While it has philosophical roots, the transformative quality of yoga comes from doing something intentionally different from what is most familiar and habitual. The yoga teachings encourage us to confront and transform the patterns that take us towards suffering. They also emphasize that nothing can be changed unless it is first brought into consciousness. This change process necessitates that we learn to dance with the feeling of awkward. Awkwardness begets a sense of discomfort and confusion. It implies that we are doing something unfamiliar. In other words, we are not stuck in our pattern. It is precisely this state of uncertainty that provides fertile ground for our evolution, personal growth, and learning.

Reading about the physiology of respiration is fascinating. *Restoring Prāṇa* is full of scientific facts from both the Vedic and Western medical traditions. However, reading, like thinking, has relatively little potency when it comes to altering behavior. The juice of the *Restoring Prāṇa* text is expressed through the practices themselves. I have my doubts that reading the book and memorizing the facts alone will impact your life to any degree. You have to apply the knowledge in an active way. Conversely, one could do these practices without knowing any of the background science and experience metamorphosis.

The SBJ is an invitation to step up and take action. I challenge you to play with the practices described, using your breath, body, and mind as your own personal laboratory. Each chapter offers a unique inquiry for your study. Through the interweave of these experiential processes you will come to understand much about your relationship to your breath, to every other system of your body, and to your mind. The SBJ offers you multiple opportunities to restructure your breathing pattern, through awareness and practice: the magic combo!

Each chapter correlates with the chapters in *Restoring Prāṇa*, opening with a brief summary of the key concepts laid out in the source text. This creates context for the practices that follow as well as a short review of major ideas. You'll find that some of the practices are more reflective, asking you to write or journal your thoughts or feelings about the breath. Others will call you to the mat and invite you to move your body in new or different ways. These practices combine breath and movement with deep intentionality to enhance your experience and understanding of both. Still other practices will ask you to track your breathing patterns over time and to chart various barometers, such as heart rate, breath rate, and breath-hold time. You may find that some of the practices resonate or reveal more to you, while colleagues or friends have a very different experience. That is to be expected. I wouldn't anticipate that you would find each and every practice to be earth-shattering. It's the culmination of information gleaned from consistent attention and activation that will fertilize your self-knowledge.

If you're the kind of person who thinks the goodies are always at the end of this kind of text, you may feel inclined to skip ahead to what you perceive as the most important or difficult processes (presumably in the last few chapters). However, I guarantee you that this workbook is not set up in that kind of format. The prāṇāyāma program created in *Restoring Prāṇa* and detailed explicitly in this workbook provides a systematic building process that emphasizes the development of awareness, *not difficulty*. If you are utilizing this workbook as the manual to the online Restore Your Prāṇa certification program, you will have an assigned mentor who will guide you through your process. They will adapt and customize it appropriately for you. If you would like to register for the online Restore Your Prāṇa certification program, please send your queries to info@essentialyogatherapy.com.

This workbook is also intended as a support for yoga teacher trainers and program directors who have been certified to teach the Restore Your Prāṇa program to others. If you are interested in becoming a certified Restore Your Prāṇa trainer, contact robin@essentialyogatherapy.com for registration details.

Awareness can neither be short-circuited nor accelerated beyond the authenticity and commitment you bring to it. Some of us are faster processors and some need more time to let an experience marinate until it is fully understood. My recommendation is that you treat each chapter as approximately a month's worth of material to digest. If you are working with the Restore Your Prāṇa online program, you will have an assigned mentor who will guide you through your process, adapting and fine-tuning it appropriately for you. If you are receiving this as part of your teacher or therapist training program, your instructor will monitor your progress and offer ideas about how you can optimize the teachings and practices to suit your learning style. If you are using this workbook as a self-guided process, I would highly recommend that you work very closely with the *Restoring Prāṇa* text. Be sure to attend to all the nuances outlined there with regard to respiratory physiology and the variable impact of changing the breath on health and mental stability. Whatever your orientation, breath retraining cannot be forced or pushed! This program is intended to be a 10–12-month process. Changing your body's chemistry requires slow percolation, with steady reinforcement. Pushing an agenda on your breath will likely backfire, causing your prāṇa to be depleted, dispersed, or distorted, rather than restored.

Notes

There are many Sanskrit terms utilized throughout this text. Sanskrit is the language of the original yoga teachings. To allow for easier flow in reading, definitions of each word will be offered the first time a term is used. There is a full glossary provided at the end of the book which also gives the pronunciation of the term.

There are online webinars available for purchase to support those who are using this as a self guided program. They are available at www.essentialyogatherapy.com/breathing-lite-and-restoring-prana.

1

THE BREATH AS A WINDOW INTO YOUR WORLD

The teachings of *Sāṁkhya* form the philosophical basis of yoga and Ayurveda. Sāṁkhya describes the manifest world—which is known as *prakṛti*—as being infused with *prāṇa*. Prāṇa represents the animating life-force. Everything known to us contains prāṇa and comprises three inherent qualities. These qualities of nature are referred to as the *guṇas* and are: activity or *rajas*, inertia or *tamas*, and light/harmony or *sattva* (see Figure 1.1).

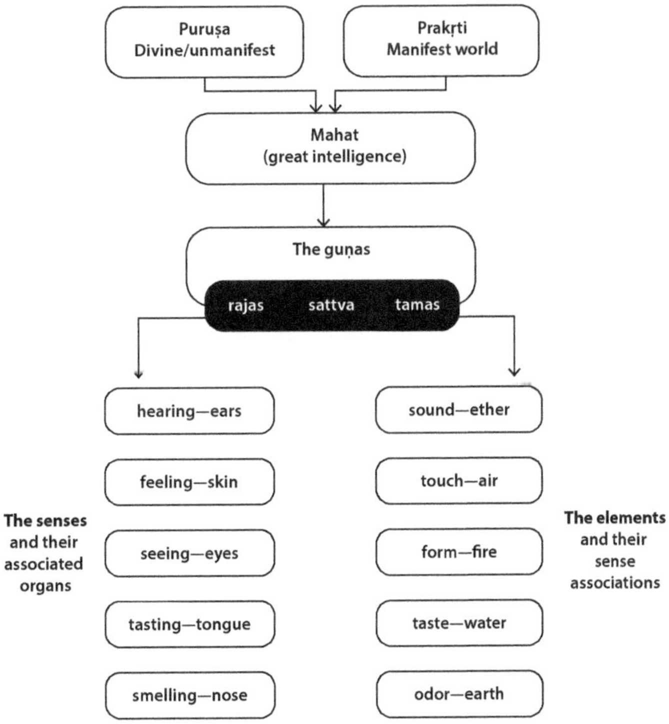

Figure 1.1 Sāṁkhya Evolution

Like the forces of nature, prāṇa within us can be agitated, stagnant, or balanced. The practices of yoga are intended to support healthy containment and restoration of our prāṇa so we can live our lives in an intelligent and conscious way. Prāṇāyāma, the fourth limb of the eight-limbed system of yoga, acts as the primary means to address our prāṇic imbalances. The original yoga texts associate prāṇāyāma with breath retention and suspension, not with taking large gulps of breath in and out. In fact, the description of inhalation and exhalation is that they are to be made subtle, to the point of near imperceptibility. In other words, to breathe with yogic intent we need to *breathe less not more*. Restraining the output and input of breath is said to increase vitality and quiet the mind.

In modern times, this concept of prāṇāyāma has been all but lost. Contemporary yoga practices often center around the perfection of posture, fortified by dramatic breathing techniques. The ancient yogis were less focused on physical prowess through the attainment of āsana. The definition of yoga offered by Patañjali's Yoga Sūtra 1.2 describes yoga as the state in which the mind has ceased its habitual swirling and resides in stillness. These teachings go on to emphasize that the link between the mind and the breath is inseparable. They specify that as the breath grows more agitated (rajas) or dull (tamas), so goes the mind and vice versa. Through prāṇāyāma we can learn to bring the breath into sattvic stillness, thus preparing the mind for deep states of meditation.

The challenge in downshifting the breath is that we often have no idea what it means to breathe lighter and less. Most breath instructions indicate that it is healthy to breathe harder and more. We'll explore the physiological misstep in this line of thinking in future chapters. The intention of this chapter is to begin the process of *svādhyāya*—or self-awareness—of your breath habit. How do you actually breathe? How often? How much does your mind impact your breath, and your breath impact your mind?

Patañjali defines the intent of yoga practice as alleviating suffering in our lives. According to the Yoga Sūtra, the *vṛttis*, or turnings of the mind, are the primary source of our self-imposed afflictions, known as the *kleśas*. Patañjali specifies three tools to activate the yogic process of changing habitual patterns that create suffering, to relieve us of the bondage of the kleśas: disciplined effort, known as *tapas*; self-awareness, or *svādhyāya*; and devotion to the highest, or *īśvarapraṇidhāna*. He calls the combination of these three *kriya yoga*, or the yoga of action, and suggests that together they offer the best possibility for inducing lasting, positive change. Each subsequent chapter of this Svādhyāya Breath Journal (SBJ) will draw heavily from this kriya yoga teaching. It forms the foundation for your breath exploration practices and transformation process.

The principal call to action in this chapter is to practice paying attention to what has been simmering below the radar of your consciousness. Habituated patterns that have formed a deep neurophysiological groove in our system are known as *saṃskāras*. Breath and thought are our most deep-seated saṃskāras, ones that we engage in throughout every day. Our breath rate hovers between 15,000 and 20,000 breaths a day. Preliminary research estimates that we think at more than double that rate, although there are no conclusive studies on an exact number. These kinds of repetitive patterns don't shift easily, or at all, if they remain unconscious. Our breathing pattern is challenging to change, precisely because it requires us to pay attention to something we mostly ignore, except in times of intense stress or physical exertion. Even as you become more aware of how you breathe, altering the breath saṃskāra can feel awkward, almost as if you are shedding your own skin. For this reason, as you cultivate your Restore Your Prāṇa practice, you'll be encouraged to build slowly and bring compassion and patience to the experience.

As your awareness grows, you will feel prepared and empowered to naturally take the next step forward in the process.

Kriya Yoga Exploration

To transform a pattern, we must be able to identify it. The process of observation described below draws on the three aspects of kriya yoga to provide insight into your breath saṃskāras. This information will help you to synthesize and utilize the information in the upcoming chapters. Ultimately, knowing yourself in this intimate way will enable you to choose the appropriate prāṇāyāma techniques in order to create practices that promote sattva. To support you in this process, I encourage you to carry your Svādhyāya Breath Journal (SBJ) with you so, like a scientist, you can observe yourself through the microscope of daily life.

Svādhyāya on the Breath

PRACTICE 1.1: DAILY ACCOUNTING

Take daily notes for several weeks, developing a beneficial habit of consistent observation of the breath and its impact on you. Make notes at various points during your daily routine, such as before or after meals, or when shifting between home and work. You may wish to note changes in the breath when a particular circumstance arises, such as when you have deadlines or events where there is more pressure. Compare and contrast those experiences with times you feel relaxed or are celebrating. Be as detailed as you can about what you notice. I recommend cultivating a serious dose of curiosity about what you will discover. Channel your inner scientist so the process is motivated by intrigue rather than imposition!

Use this space to journal your day-by-day observances. Keep your answers brief, noting only what is coming up for you in your svādhyāya process. In true yoga style, apply a generous dollop of non-judgment to your observation process. On the days when you forget, just note that, as this will also inform your growing self-understanding. Your observations will form the basis for the rest of the practices in this section.

EXAMPLE

Week 1—July 2019

Day 6 Date 7/05/19 Overall observances of breath:

My breath today feels tight in my chest. I didn't sleep well last night and the house has been chaotic with all the preparations for our upcoming trip. I found myself taking big sighs and holding my breath at times.

Week 1 Month ___________ Year ___________

Day 1 Date ___________ Overall observances of breath

___

___

___

Day 2 Date ___________ Overall observances of breath

___

___

___

Day 3 Date ___________ Overall observances of breath

___

___

___

Day 4 Date ___________ Overall observances of breath

___

___

___

Day 5 Date ___________ Overall observances of breath

___

___

___

Day 6 Date ___________ Overall observances of breath

___

___

___

Day 7 Date ___________ Overall observances of breath

___

___

___

Week 2 Month ____________ Year ____________

Day 1 Date ____________ Overall observances of breath

____

____

____

Day 2 Date ____________ Overall observances of breath

____

____

____

Day 3 Date ____________ Overall observances of breath

____

____

____

Day 4 Date ____________ Overall observances of breath

____

____

____

Day 5 Date ____________ Overall observances of breath

____

____

____

Day 6 Date ____________ Overall observances of breath

____

____

____

Day 7 Date ____________ Overall observances of breath

____

____

____

Week 3 Month ___________ Year ___________

Day 1 Date ___________ Overall observances of breath

____

____

____

Day 2 Date ___________ Overall observances of breath

____

____

____

Day 3 Date ___________ Overall observances of breath

____

____

____

Day 4 Date ___________ Overall observances of breath

____

____

____

Day 5 Date ___________ Overall observances of breath

____

____

____

Day 6 Date ___________ Overall observances of breath

____

____

____

Day 7 Date ___________ Overall observances of breath

____

____

____

Week 4 Month ____________ Year ____________

Day 1 Date ____________ Overall observances of breath

____

____

____

Day 2 Date ____________ Overall observances of breath

____

____

____

Day 3 Date ____________ Overall observances of breath

____

____

____

Day 4 Date ____________ Overall observances of breath

____

____

____

Day 5 Date ____________ Overall observances of breath

____

____

____

Day 6 Date ____________ Overall observances of breath

____

____

____

Day 7 Date ____________ Overall observances of breath

____

____

____

PRACTICE 1.2: THE BREATH AND THE GUṆAS

Use the spaces below to record your reflections on any or all of the following:

- As you observe your regular breathing habit (saṃskāra), note what patterns in relationship to the guṇas are most prominent.
  - What are some events or circumstances that cause your breath to take on rajasic characteristics, such as rapid, shallow, erratic, or loud? What else do you notice about how you feel in those moments?

    ____

    ____

    ____

    ____

  - What are some events or circumstances that cause your breath to take on tamasic characteristics, such as withheld, restricted, tight, and heavy? What else do you notice about how you feel in those moments?

    ____

    ____

    ____

    ____

  - What are some events or circumstances that cause your breath to take on sattvic characteristics, such as smooth, quiet at rest, steady, easeful, and light? What else do you notice about how you feel in those moments?

    ____

    ____

    ____

    ____

- In reflecting on your responses above, please note the predominant guṇa activating the mind at these times as well. Is there a correlation (e.g. breath rajasic—mind rajasic, or otherwise)?

  ____

  ____

  ____

  ____

- What senses are stimulated during times of rajasic or tamasic breath patterns—for example, seeing or hearing something that stimulates you or shuts you down, such as a movie, a news report, or a particular smell that excites you, such as baking cookies?

- How does the experience of sattvic breathing differ from rajasic and tamasic patterns? What do you notice about how this sensory experience compares to the others?

- How do your senses impact the breath and mind?

PRACTICE 1.3: THE BREATH AND THE KLEŚAS

Patañjali defines the kleśas as the seeds of suffering. They are considered to be afflictions or impediments to practice. He states that ignorance, ego, attachment, aversion, and fear fuel much of what creates internal and external struggle. The practices of kriya yoga described above are intended to subdue or loosen the knots of constriction that are formed by the kleśas. Read through the list of the kleśas below and consider and note how these states of mind impact your breath.

- **avidya:** Ignorance.

- **asmitā:** I-am-ness. The awareness of oneself as a distinct being.

- **raga:** Interpreted in most texts as attachment, raga speaks to our tendency to become attached to the experiences that we consider pleasant or pleasurable.

- **dveṣa:** Aversion.

- **abhinevesha:** Fear, ultimately the fear of death.

In your observation, note which of the kleśas are fanned by the acceleration, constriction, or arrhythmic quality of your breath. As you observe your breath through the kleśas, what patterns emerge? For example, you may notice that when you're in a state of raga, of want or desire, your breath is more rajasic.

PRACTICE 1.4: YOUR BREATH IN ĀSANA

- How would you describe the quality of your breath when you practice āsana (rajasic, tamasic, or sattvic)?

- Can you practice āsana in a way that is more sattvic (quiet, light, rhythmic, easeful)? How does the felt sense of your experience change during and after practice when you bring attention to maintaining a sattvic breath? What do you notice?

- Try applying this same awareness and strategy to forms of exercise (e.g. walking, cycling, swimming). What do you notice in the process?

Tapas with the Breath

PRACTICE 1.5: SAṂSKĀRA TRANSFORMATION

After you take some time to observe the connections between your natural breath, your mind, and your activities, choose one arena to begin to gently initiate restraint. For example, if you notice that you huff and puff while going up the hill on your morning walk, try slowing down, closing your mouth, and maintaining a more sattvic breath quality that is quiet, light, rhythmic, and easeful. Or perhaps you notice your breath getting agitated while driving. Develop a practice of breathing lightly while in the car and steadying the flow.

Start with one area where you identify a consistent tendency for your breath to be arrhythmic, heavy, or chaotic. Practice transforming just that single pattern before attempting to broaden your focus to other areas of your life.

Use the space below to write your overall reflections on this process over the course of several weeks to a month.

EXAMPLE

Name of pattern: Hard, mouth breathing when walking.

How often do you observe this? 5x a week when walking my dog.

Approach to change: Walking more slowly and keeping my mouth closed when I become breathless.

Consistency of practice: 2–3x a week I am able to do this, except when I'm rushing off to work and don't have time.

Reflections or results of practice: It's super-hard to slow down. When I do, it actually feels better to breathe with my mouth closed and I feel calmer. My mouth isn't as dry and I don't need to drink as much water when I get home. At the same time, moving that slowly feels like I'm not getting as much of a workout. I also am aware of how impatient I am to get on to the rest of my day. Sometimes it's super-frustrating.

Name of pattern: ______________________________

How often do you observe this? ______________________________

Approach to change: ______________________________

Consistency of practice: ______________________________

Reflections or results of practice: ______________________________

____

____

____

____

____

____

____

____

PRACTICE 1.6: BREATH IN ĀSANA AND PRĀṆĀYĀMA PRACTICE—CHANGING OUR SĀDHANĀ PRACTICE

When you are practicing āsana and/or prāṇāyāma, practice breathing as the yogis suggest:

- Through the nose.
- Sattvic (light, easeful).
- Subtle.
- Abdominal-diaphragmatic, maintaining passivity in the muscles of the chest.
- Focus on the external space just outside your nostrils and reduce the volume of breath as it travels outward upon exhale. You can gauge this by holding your index finger under your nose routinely and monitoring how much breath you feel passing over your finger. Can you lighten the flow so it's barely detectable? How difficult is it to maintain that level throughout your practice?
- Focus on the internal space within your body as you breathe. Visualize the breath permeating your cells and the interstitial space. Picture yourself infusing them with prāṇa.
- Begin to develop the pause after inhale/exhale. Hold for 2, 4, 6, upward to 10 seconds. Notice your relative comfort level with these two phases of the breath. What do you notice when you hold after the inhale? What do you notice when you hold after the exhale?

In the space below, document your experience of doing this tapas practice during āsana and prāṇāyāma. Use the prompts to help you describe your observation.

- What do you notice about the relative ease or challenge of doing this?

- How does this practice challenge the breath saṃskāras you've developed through prior practice and study of yoga?

- What do you notice about your attachments—if any—to the idea or experience of taking a bigger breath, sighing, and/or breathing through your mouth?

- Note your observations about how shifting your breath impacts the mind, the senses, the grip of the kleśas (afflictions), and your overall self-awareness.

Īśvarapraṇidhāna with the Breath

PRACTICE 1.7: REMEMBERING THE DIVINE—MANTRA AND THE BREATH

There are numerous ways to raise spiritual awareness. Linking connection to Īśvara (the Divine, Source, the Highest) with the constancy of the breath enables us to practice anywhere, any time. One powerful tool, the practice of mantra, can be used like a touchstone in times of stress or when you recognize you are out of alignment with what is highest for you. In fact, this is the intention of mantra: to transcend the ordinary mind and transform the vṛttis. Mantra recitation can be nourished through either daily prāṇāyāma or āsana practice.

Here are just a few suggestions for the use of silent mantra to build your connection to the Divine via the breath. Choose one or experiment with a few and notice the effect:

- Silently recite a word or prayer (a mantra) with each exhalation during your āsana and/or prāṇāyāma practice. Choose a word that expresses a quality you would like to cultivate, such as Light, Love, Joy, or Peace.
- Use one of the yamas as a focus for the breath.The yamas, or ethical principles of yoga, provide a wonderful foundation for spiritual practice. The five yamas (listed below) define the first limb of the eight-limbed system of yoga detailed by Patañjali in the second chapter of the Yoga Sūtras. The yamas reflect our relationship to self and others, calling us to restrain our base instincts and elevate our thoughts and actions to better serve our community with compassion and care. Experiment with reciting the yama of your choice silently, with inhale, exhale, or both. Note the effect on your state of mind.

YAMA: THE FIRST LIMB OF YOGA

- **ahimsā:** Non-violence, cultivation of compassion and empathy for others
- **satya:** Truthful communication; refraining from gossip, speaking with ahimsa
- **asteya:** Integrity in action; not taking what has not been offered to us
- **brahmacharya:** Conservation of energy; abstaining from actions that deplete us or infringe on others
- **aparigrahā:** Living simply with what we need rather than hoarding what we want

- Use the word "sattva" as a reminder to keep the breath steady and calm, and as a reminder of the illuminative light within you.
- Choose a soothing word or phrase from your own religious or spiritual liturgy that is meaningful to you. Repeat it silently, as suggested above. For example, with each exhale, silently repeat one of these: Jesus is with me; let go, let God; inshallah; b'shalom; om shanti.

Use the space below to reflect upon how your īśvarapraṇidhāna practice or use of mantra has impacted your breath, your mind, your awareness, and any other aspect of your being. How does mantra impact your breath? What changes do you notice in your mind or awareness with use of mantra?

PRACTICE 1.8: MANTRA AND BREATH IN ACTION

Combine your mantra practice with your tapas practice. For example, based on the practices above, you might silently recite your mantra while walking or driving, in order to directly impact the quality and flow of the breath. How does reciting your mantra affect your experience of the breath and mind and the relationship between them?

Use the space below to reflect upon how your ISP practice or use of mantra has impacted your breath, your mind, your awareness, and any other aspect of your being. What was your mantra? What was your tapas practice? What happened when you used mantra in combination with your tapas practice? What would you most like to remember about the effects of this combination?

2

THE FIVE WINDS AND YOUR ENERGY BANK ACCOUNT

In Chapter 1, you examined your breath habits and began to develop svādhyāya—self-awareness of how your breath changes as you live your life. Through the tapas process, you experimented with disciplined practice to alter your breath pattern by shifting it intentionally to become more reserved and steady. You used mantra to bring a more devotional or spiritual meaning to your change process and reflected on how that impacted the internal felt sense of your breath and mind. All of this is moving you in the direction of prāṇāyāma as it was originally intended. Prāṇa is subtle. Practice requires you to attune yourself to "listen" or "sense" at more subtle frequencies.

The ancient yogis used prāṇāyāma as a practice of breath restraint in order to govern prāṇa, elevate awareness, and direct attention. However, their world was more prāṇically balanced, with fewer demands than most of us experience day to day. Nowadays, fundamental resources such as water, air, and soil have been tainted by man-made pollutants. Additionally, our lifestyle is faster, full of constant interaction and sensory bombardment. We literally have to "retreat" from our daily lives in order to experience a moment of stillness and silence. The more prāṇa that is gobbled up by wrangling all that chaos, the less we have available to support our health.

Breath was used by the yogis as a "diagnostic" tool for assessing vitality. Improper breathing was commensurate with health concerns and mental instability. While many of the intense breath ratios referenced in the original texts make sense for the conditions of that time, prāṇāyāma practices today need to be adapted and titrated appropriately according to our environmental, cultural, and individual circumstances. This requires a high degree of calibration to ensure that our prāṇāyāma practices facilitate our health in these complex modern times, rather than stressing our already strained system.

The Guṇas and the Elements

As stated in Chapter 1, prakṛti is made up of the guṇas. The elements—earth, wind, fire, air, and space—are derived from the guṇas and are infused with prāṇa. They exist within us and formulate the world around us. The Ayurvedic dośas are elemental composites that draw on the primary qualities associated with each of the element (see Figure 2.1). The dośas are vata, pitta, and kapha. Imbalance in the dośas indicates prāṇic imbalance requiring our attention. Just like us, the prāṇa in the world is not doshically stable. Seasonal changes impact our health, and now significant elemental shifts in climate are affecting the planet universally. As the environment is thrown out of balance, our physiological and mental health are being affected. Our yoga practices, including prāṇāyāma, can help return us to a more sattvic state. This in turn can support our living in a more harmonious way with the planet at large.

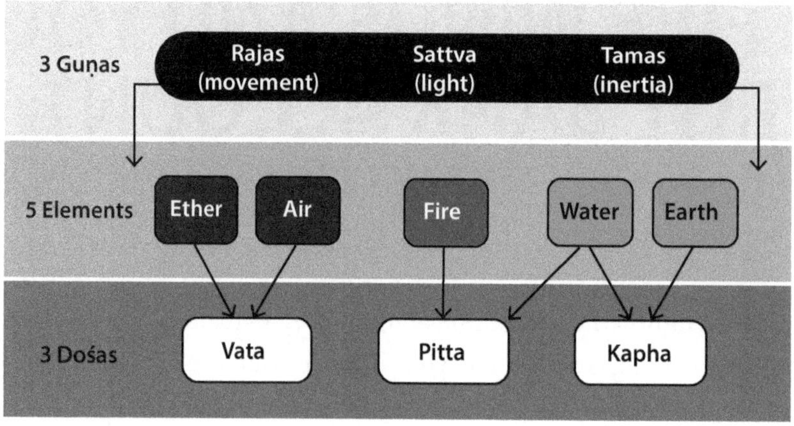

Figure 2.1 The Guṇas, the Elements, and the Dośas

The Panchamaya—the Five Dimensions

According to the Vedic teachings, we are multi-dimensional, comprising a physical, vital, mental, emotional, and spiritual component. This teaching of the five dimensions is known as the *panchamaya*, or five inseparable facets of our prakṛti. In many yoga lineages, the panchamaya are referred to as the *maya koshas*. While these five dimensions are often depicted like nesting dolls within one another (see Figure 2.2), they really interrelate and each sphere impacts the others, more like an interactive Venn diagram (see Figure 2.3).

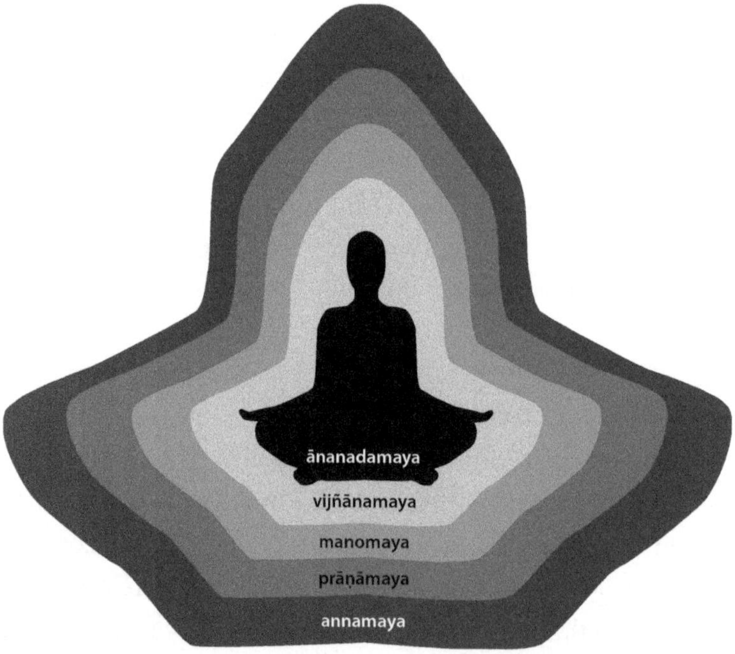

Figure 2.2 The Panchamaya

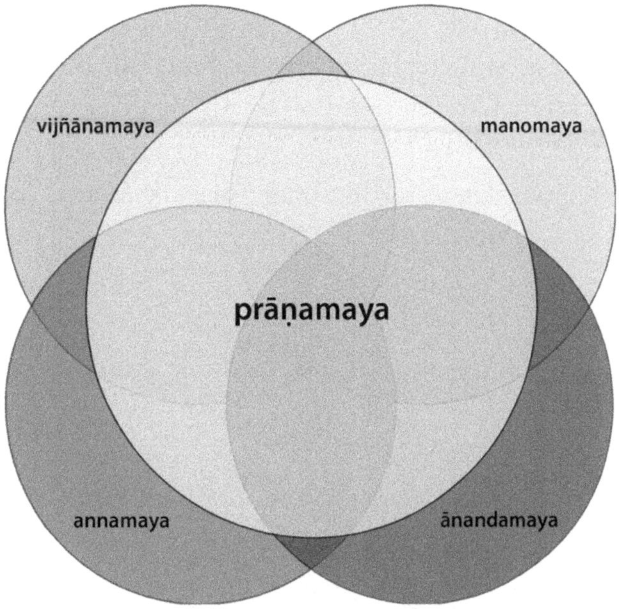

Figure 2.3 The Panchamaya through Prāṇamaya

THE PANCHAMAYA

- **annamaya:** The food or physical dimension; considered the musculoskeletal dimension, it is composed of the five elements: earth, water, air, fire, ether.
- **prāṇamaya:** The prāṇic or vital dimension that houses the subtle body. The prāṇamaya is intimately related to the breath, physiological function, and health. It is made up of the five winds or vāyus.
- **manomaya:** The dimension of the mind and the senses. The manomaya knows the world through comparison and relativity; one thing is bigger, hotter, better than another. The five senses and the mind together provide internal and external information that impact our perception of the world and sustain us in dualistic thinking.
- **vijñānamaya:** The dimension of wisdom; the root "jña" refers to inner knowledge. Vijñānamaya is a deeper level of mind than manomaya. It is linked to our subconscious beliefs, cultural attitudes, and patterns that have been transmitted generationally. Vijñānamaya also provides the seat of creativity, original thought, and the wisdom of discernment.
- **ānandamaya:** The spiritual heart of our being. The word "ānanda" refers to the inherent quality of expansiveness within us. This is the joy of connection, of belonging, of devotion and openhearted love. At the level of ānandamaya, the mind is able to move beyond duality and rejoin, relink with puruṣa, the Divine.

The Prāṇamaya and the Panchavāyus—the Five Winds

The prāṇamaya, the energy dimension, is made up of five types of prāṇas, or winds, called *vāyus.* These winds correlate with the breath, the elements of air and space, and the Ayurvedic dośas of vata. Like the wind, they are rajasic (active), subtle, and pervasive. They move us and move through us in unseen yet palpable ways. Each vāyu governs a particular aspect of what we might think of as our physiology and mental activity. In Ayurvedic medicine the relative balance of the vāyus is used to ascertain health and disease. An understanding of the vāyus supports our study of prāṇāyāma and the link between the breath and our health. This concept is fundamental to both yoga and Ayurveda. Figure 2.4 illustrates the panchavāyus and their directional flow of movement.

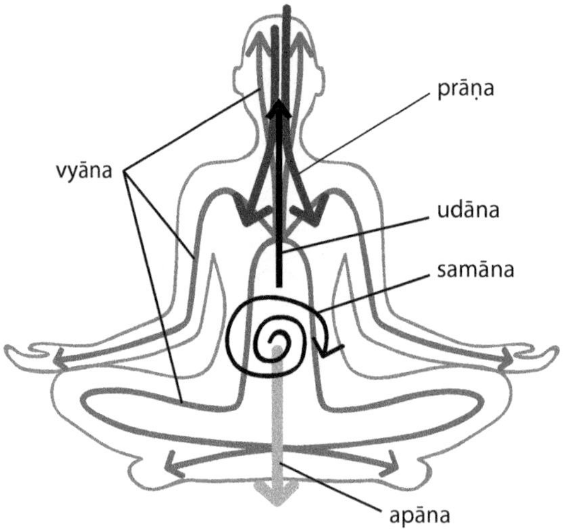

Figure 2.4 The Panchavāyus

THE PANCHAVĀYUS—THE FIVE WINDS

- **prāṇa:** Incoming energy via the senses; movement is down and in. Governs everything we take in, including air, water, food, sights, sounds, taste, smells, touch, information, ideas, and experiences. Breath: Directs inhalation, the taking in of oxygen.
- **apāna:** Outgoing energy in the way of waste, negativity; movement is down and out. Governs defecation, urination, perspiration, menstruation, ejaculation, and even the process of birth. It also governs the release of negative emotions, sensory experiences, and thoughts. Breath: Directs exhalation in terms of the release of excess CO_2.
- **samāna:** Energy of digestion; centered in belly, the seat of agni, the digestive fire. Governs digestion of nutrients, thoughts, emotions, ideas, spiritual experience. Breath: Supports perfusion in the lungs, greater absorption of O_2 into the bloodstream. Correlates with retention of breath after inhale.
- **vyāna:** Energy of assimilation/absorption; movement is outward from samānavayu into the body. Governs circulation via the blood and plasma; neurotransmission; and endocrine secretions. Breath: Supports cellular respiration via the dispersion of O_2 through the bloodstream into the tissues; metabolism; and production of CO_2. Correlates with suspension of breath after exhale.

- **udāna:** Energy of upliftment, transformation, and growth, physical as well as spiritual. Upward and forward-moving wind. Governs growth, the ability to stand, speak, step forward, the expression of enthusiasm, positivity, singing, laughter, vomiting, belching, coughing. Breath: Directs the movement of exhalation.

The Vāyus, the Breath, and Our "Energy Bank Account" (EBA)

Just as there can be too much food or anything else, too much breath can be burdensome for our system. Like the earth's atmosphere, fluctuations in oxygen and carbon dioxide levels in our bodies can have devastating consequences. In our body, the proper balance between these two formative gases must be maintained at appropriate levels to sustain our health. The breath acts as the primary driver of the chemical reactions that maintain the vāyus in homeostasis, or balance. The quality and quantity of our breath, and rate at which we breathe in and out, have a significant impact on how we ultimately feel. Respiration actively regulates our ability to digest, assimilate, and eliminate. How well we synthesize what we take in is directly reflected in udāna, in what comes up and out of us (e.g. joy, rage, fear, desire).

Understanding the Vāyus in Daily Life

If we gulp air in with big gasps, it's as if every day is a Thanksgiving feast. In essence we are consuming 5000 calories of air when 2000 is sufficient. Likewise, if we are constantly talking, sighing, yawning, coughing, and snoring, it's as if we had a case of the "runs," depleting our reserves of carbon dioxide. We need the appropriate balance of O_2 and CO_2 in order to maintain our health. Breathing lightly in and out nourishes us without taxing our system and maintains our gas equilibrium in healthy parameters. (These ideas will be detailed in Chapters 3 and 4.) The practice of prāṇāyāma evolved out of this keen recognition, which is why the yogis cautioned us to retain prāṇa. They emphasized kumbhāka—that is, both breath retention and suspension. Kumbhāka provide periods of rest to allow for greater perfusion and assimilation of O_2 and CO_2 between breaths.

In the truest sense, prāṇāyāma is akin to going on an "air diet." This is what is required for many of us to get our prāṇamaya back to homeostasis. The functioning of the panchavāyus depends on good oxygenation of the tissues. As you explore the effect of over-breathing in the upcoming chapters on physiology, you'll come to understand why proper oxygenation does not come from front-loading the system with an onslaught of air. The secret of vitality, known as vīrya, lies in our capacity to utilize small amounts of oxygen efficiently. That requires balance throughout the prāṇamaya.

Assessing your own energy system through the lens of the panchavāyus is a fundamental process that should precede serious prāṇāyāma practice. To ascertain whether the practice is serving to restore your prāṇa or depleting you further, it's important to get a baseline understanding of your energetic starting point. The process of taking inventory of your Energy Bank Account (EBA) is much like balancing your check book. You make deposits (prāṇavayu) and withdrawals (apānavayu), and either you have reserves or you don't. If you take out too much or don't invest in your future (samāna and vyāna vāyus), you'll end up in the red.

The practices in this section offer a way of facilitating an EBA assessment. I suggest you use them as a baseline for your prāṇāyāma practice. They can reveal to you where and on what level of the vāyus you are losing prāṇa. They'll also give clues as to where your prāṇic reservoir needs to be sealed or purified.

You may find it useful to revisit the questions in these practices many times over the course of this program. Use them as a means to gauge how your breath practice is supporting your health. I require both my yoga therapy trainees and many of my therapeutic clients to go through this process, particularly those with auto-immune conditions. All have found it to be revelatory.

Through contemplation of their EBA, many of my chronic fatigue clients have come to recognize that they don't allow themselves time for digestion and assimilation, time to pause to refuel. They find that this connect-the-dots process reveals cause and effect between a life-long habit (saṃskāra) of driving themselves to do (rajas) and ending up in bed, exhausted (tamas). Often their healing accelerates significantly as they learn to pace each day and live more sattvically—in balance/harmony. This means allowing time to rest, digest, and recover before the next errand or social event. It may also require learning to say, "No," to simplify their life, in order to shift their health in a positive direction.

PRACTICE 2.1: ASSESSING YOUR EBA

Consider the reflective questions below in measurements of a typical day, week, or month. You may find it useful to break the time frame down into even smaller increments, such as morning versus afternoon, or hour by hour.

- What do you take in? Consider all that you take in through the senses and the mind, including information and education, over the course of day, a week, a month.

EXAMPLE

Most days I listen to the morning news. I engage in conversations with my family and co-workers. I eat 2+ meals and several small snacks (mostly protein and veggies, but some ice cream 2x a week too ☺). I like to listen to music on the way home from work or podcasts when I work out. In the evenings, I watch an hour or two of TV, or spend an hour on Facebook. On the weekends, my husband and I tend to get together with friends, and eat more, drink more (alcohol, maybe several glasses of wine or a couple of cocktails). Some nights I meditate for 15 minutes before bed (taking in silence and stillness).

- What energy do you put out in the course of a day, a week, a month?

____

____

____

EXAMPLE

Most days I get up at 6, get my two kids ready for school (ages 10 & 12), make them breakfast, pack lunches and drive them to school before work. I tend to our three dogs and make breakfast for my husband if he's not traveling. I go to work where I am a teacher and spend the day with 10 second-graders. If I don't have a faculty or parent conference, I pick up the kids after school, go grocery shopping (sometimes I have other errands as well, like taking the kids to piano lessons or sports practices). When I get home I make dinner, help the kids with their homework; sometimes I have to do preparatory work for the next day at school. My husband often wants to share about his day and so I try to be available for him. My mom has a heart condition so 1–2x a week I stop over to see her and make sure she and my dad are okay. I often have to pick up prescriptions for the two of them and negotiate with the nurse who sees to them. I try and work out 3x a week, get to my Sat. morning yoga class, and I try to take my dogs for a walk every day, but sometimes I'm just too tired and can't get out the door. Weekends the kids have soccer and baseball games, so I'm often carpooling other kids as well.

PRACTICE 2.2: YOUR EBA CLOSE UP AND PERSONAL

Keeping in mind the general reflection from your answers above, dive into some more specifics. There is no right or wrong way of doing this assessment. For instance, going for a walk for some of you may fall into the prāṇa category—for example, taking in air, and the sensory components of trees, plants, sounds, and information from signs. For others it may be considered an act of udāna, as you are putting out energy, especially if you're walking and talking with friends. Other may consider walking to be a time of digestion, or samāna—for example, contemplating the form of a flower, the spirit of the trees, thinking over something that happened earlier. The intention is for you to consider how your daily life experiences impact you prāṇically, and to approximate how much prāṇa you are generating/expending in each of the vāyus.

- What percentage of your day is spent taking in? (estimate, e.g. 40%) __________
- What percentage of your day is spent giving and doing? (estimate, e.g. 60%) __________
- What percentage of your day is spent digesting experiences, food, ideas, sensory input? (estimate, e.g. based on the above calculations, 0%) __________

- What is the quality of what you are consuming or taking in (quality of food and information)?

___

___

___

- How would you characterize the pace at which you move from one activity to the next? How often do you schedule rest or pauses? How often do you have open or unscheduled days?

___

___

___

- Reflect on how much time you leave for quiet and stillness between experiences in order to digest fully. Do you find yourself caught in the busy-ness saṃskāra, chronically filling each moment with activity?

___

___

___

- How often do you find yourself doing one task while planning, strategizing, or thinking about another task? What is your process for balancing others' experiences against your own personal truth? Are you easily swayed by the opinions or beliefs of others regarding what is right for you?

___

___

___

- What are you able to let go of, and what do you cling to? Think in terms of ideas, beliefs, relationships, even spiritual aspirations.

___

___

___

- How do your beliefs both limit you and propel you towards growth?

 ____

 ____

 ____

- How much time do you spend nurturing your sense of joy, spirit, soul?

 ____

 ____

 ____

- When you speak, what do you choose to talk about? Do your words elevate the conversation, criticize, or simply take up space?

 ____

 ____

 ____

- What's the nature of your vṛttis (mind waves or fluctuations) as you examine the inner dialogues you keep with yourself? Do the vṛttis accumulate around a particular set of topics? Are they rajasic, tamasic, or sattvic in nature?

 ____

 ____

 ____

PRACTICE 2.3: THE OBSTACLES TO PRACTICE

The nine obstacles (antarāyāh) that interfere with practice and progress reflect common ways in which prāṇamaya imbalance may be displayed:

- **vyādhi:** Disease, illness, sickness
- **styāna:** Inefficiency, mental dullness
- **samśāya:** Indecision, doubt, skepticism
- **pramāda:** Carelessness, negligence, lack of interest
- **ālasaya:** Sloth, laziness
- **avirati:** Sensuality, craving
- **bhrānti darśana:** False or distorted perception

- **alabdhabhūmikatva:** Failing to meet the goals of practice
- **anavasthitatvāni:** Inability to maintain inner stability once attained.

The teaching from yoga is that chaotic or hard breathing and mental agitation are symptomatic of the antarāyāh. As you reflect on your prāṇamaya and your EBA, what obstacles are most prevalent in your life currently?

What connections do you see between your EBA, the obstacles, and your breath? How do you breathe when the obstacles present themselves?

PRACTICE 2.4: KRIYA YOGA THROUGH THE VAYUS

Once you've gone through these prāṇamaya questions, go back through the kriya yoga entries in your SBJ from Chapter 1. What can you observe about the interweave of your breath, your mind, the vāyus, and your lifestyle choices? What are the emerging patterns? Are there ways in which you channel your energy that feed into the saṃskāras that you identified in the first chapter? If you approach your āsana, prāṇāyāma, exercise, driving, and so on with the intention of balancing your vāyus, what changes in that process?

3

BREATHING BASICS: RESPIRATION 101

Chapters 1 and 2 provided a backdrop for your understanding of the teachings of yoga that relate to prāṇāyāma. I hope they instigated an exploration into your allocation of energy as it relates to the breath, your health, and your state of mind. We turn now to respiratory physiology to examine functional and dysfunctional breathing from a Western scientific perspective. This topic has three aspects to it: biochemical, biomechanical, and psychosocial. In these next two chapters we'll examine the biochemical aspect. The information and practices relayed in Chapters 3 and 4 support one another and can be completed together during a four-to-six-week period.

The Truth about Oxygenation

Breathing is fundamentally about oxygenating the cells of the body. A proper balance between oxygen (O_2) and carbon dioxide (CO_2) needs to be maintained in order for this to happen efficiently. The process of respiration is complex and enacted in three tiers:

- **Tier one—ventilation:** What we refer to as breathing is only the first tier, and is known as ventilation. Once we inhale, the air is drawn into the lungs and an exchange of gases takes place. This transpires through the alveoli, the little grape-like sacs at the ends of the bronchioles in the lungs (see Figure 3.1).

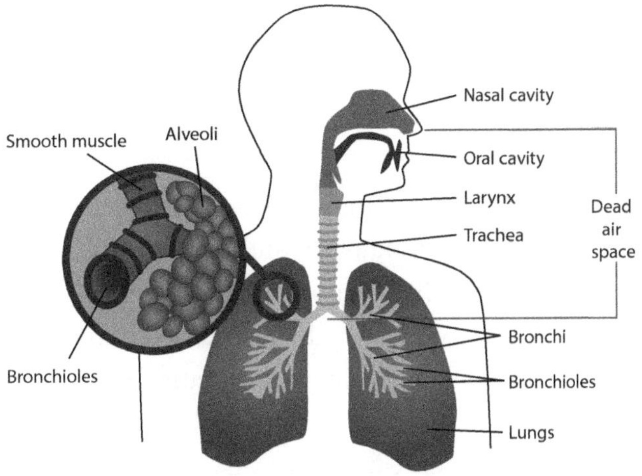

Figure 3.1 The Respiratory Tract

- **Tier two—perfusion:** The arterial and venous systems perfuse the capillaries (tiny blood vessels), feeding the alveoli CO_2 from the body, while picking up O_2 from the lungs (see Figure 3.2). Hemoglobin (red blood cells) carries the O_2 that's been taken into the lungs through the arterial system, delivering it to the tissues.

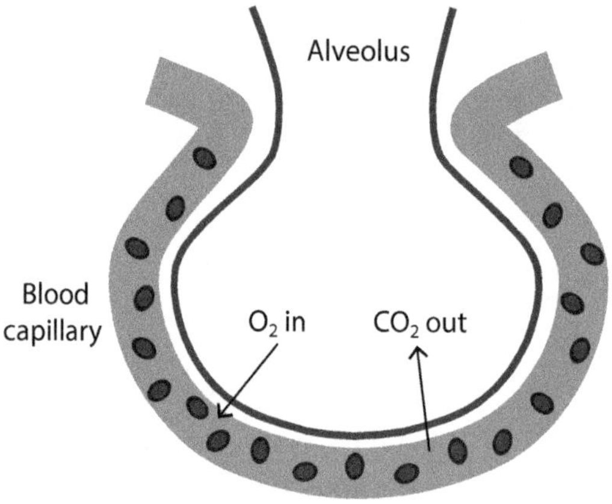

Figure 3.2 Gas Exchange through the Alveolus

- **Tier three—cellular respiration:** This tier involves the exchange of oxygen and CO_2 within the individual cells of the body, and is commonly known as oxygenation. It is cellular respiration that produces adenosine triphosphate (ATP), the organic molecule that drives many of our vital processes and gives us energy. ATP has been equated to our internal battery power keeping us energized. Oxygen fuels this process and CO_2 is a metabolic by-product of it. Excess CO_2 is released with exhalation. Ventilation (tier one) and perfusion (tier two) support cellular respiration (tier three).

A challenge we often encounter when initiating a breathing practice is the overriding myth that in order to be well oxygenated we need to breathe more. In reality, the issue is a matter of efficiency, not quantity. Breathing harder does not increase oxygenation; in fact, in people with good lung function it does the opposite. The actual amount of breath that we move through our lungs each minute, called minute volume, is calculated by multiplying our respiratory rate (breaths per minute) by our tidal volume (how much air we inhale and exhale per breath). Normal respiratory rate ranges between 8 and 12 breaths per minute, and tidal volume averages five liters per minute. When minute volume is within this range, our ability to absorb oxygen into the tissues of our body (cellular respiration) is supported. Mental and physical vitality and stability reflect a well-oxygenated system.

If CO_2 levels drop in the bloodstream, as can happen with sustained heavy breathing patterns, O_2 will bond more tightly to hemoglobin, and delivery into the tissues is then diminished (see Figure 3.3). This is due to what is known as the Bohr effect, named for the physician who discovered the phenomenon. When O_2 doesn't release into the cells, production of ATP is lowered, which may translate into muscle aches, fatigue, lethargy, brain fog, and anxiety, as well as myriad other systemic problems. Breathing harder tends to exacerbate the problem by dropping CO_2 levels even further. Ultimately, we can't get more oxygen into our body than is available in the atmosphere; however, the more we breathe, the more CO_2 is drained from our system.[1]

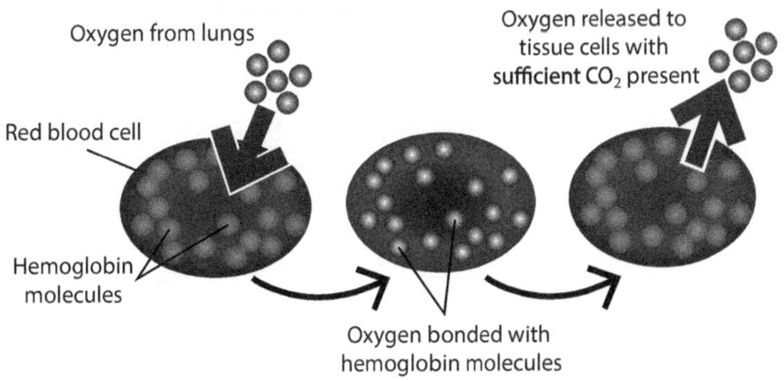

Figure 3.3 The Bohr Effect

In addition to supporting good oxygenation, CO_2 regulates pH. The pH scale is the means by which we measure the relative acid–alkaline levels in the body, with neutral being slightly alkaline (at around 7.4 when measured in morning urine or using saliva strips; see Figure 3.4). Breathing too much can compromise the acid–alkaline balance of our blood, making us vulnerable to disease. Our autonomic nervous system (ANS)—the part of our brain that regulates breathing, heart rate, digestion, and so on—is highly attuned to fluctuations in our CO_2 levels because CO_2 and pH have a symbiotic relationship. When we breathe less, pH drops; when we breathe more, it increases. Our pH needs to be consistently maintained between 7.35 and 7.45 in order for us to be healthy.

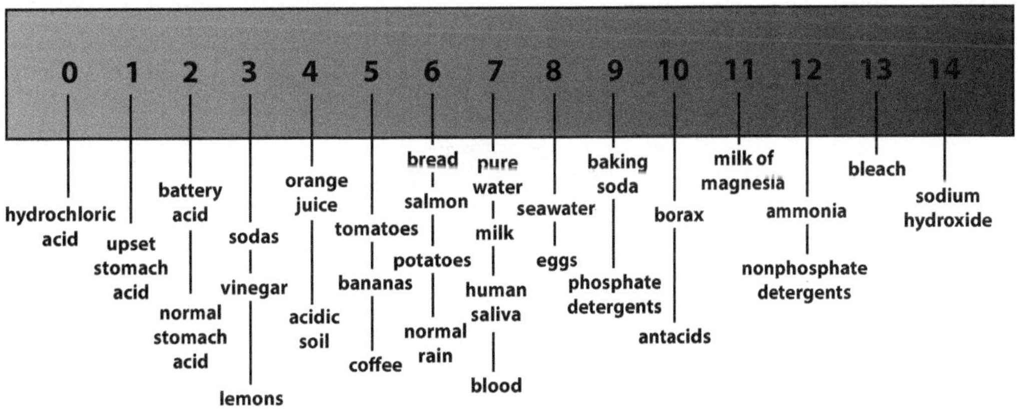

Figure 3.4 The pH Scale (Approximate Figures)

When pH fluctuates even slightly outside this narrow range for a period of time, we experience symptoms of dis-ease. If pH drops to 6 or raises to 8, we're dead (see Figure 3.5). Unlike oxygen levels, which are determined by external factors, CO_2 is a by-product of our own metabolism, making it a dependable self-regulatory gas.[2] If CO_2 drops even 1 mmHg (mmHg = millimeters of pressure) the ANS will prompt us to breathe more. Within a few breaths our pH will be back in balance. This subtle oscillation happens throughout the day without our conscious awareness and maintains our health.

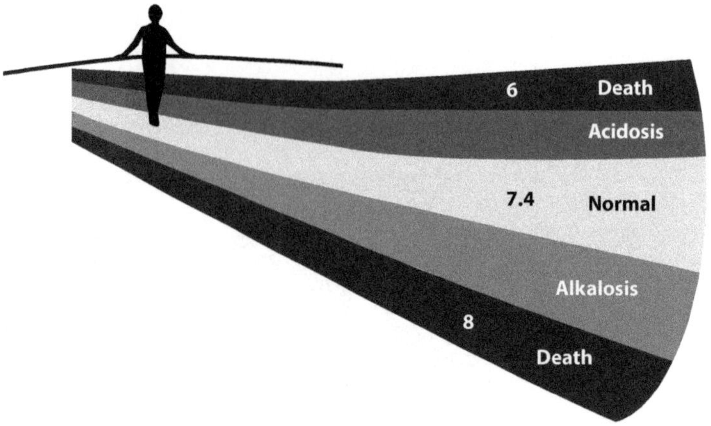

Figure 3.5 The Delicate pH Balance of Life

The medulla oblongata is the part of the brain that regulates our ANS and signals how much and how often we breathe (see Figure 3.6). The medulla acts as a kind of breathing thermostat and sets our minute volume based on how we breathe *most* of the time. As stated above, it is attuned to minor shifts in CO_2 levels. Once established, it is difficult to significantly change minute volume, because any persistent alteration in CO_2 will impact pH. As long as our breathing pattern is normal, homeostasis is maintained. However, in the case of long-term stress, chronic pain, or illness, we may develop a habit of breathing at a higher than normal minute volume. Over time, pH will shift accordingly to accommodate the lower levels of CO_2. This locks us into the new breathing pattern, one not supportive of homeostasis. Our system will then become more vulnerable to stressors. Once the big breathing habit is established, it's a bit of a vicious cycle: The more we breathe, the more we feel the need to breathe. Ironically, feeling chronically breathless or as if you're not getting enough air may actually be a reflection that you're breathing too much!

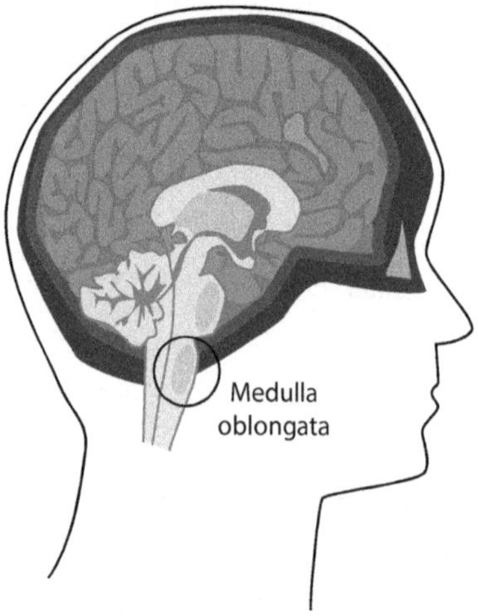

Figure 3.6 The Medulla Oblongata

When CO_2 is within a normal range, one can volitionally hold one's breath after exhalation for 30–40 seconds without signs of stress or strain. All breath-retraining processes, including prāṇāyāma, manipulate minute volume by altering rate, volume, or both in order to shift our chemistry. When successful, breathing becomes light (more subtle) and there is less sense of urgency to take big or frequent breaths. Overall, one experiences a greater ease and relaxation with the pauses between breaths.

To effectively reinforce the new minute volume, and change the set point in the medulla, multiple sessions of practice per day are required. The original teachings of yoga recommended prāṇāyāma practice four times a day. Significant kumbhāka, or breath holds of progressively increasing lengths, were a critical part of the practice. These days, prāṇāyāma (when practiced at all) is usually performed once a day, either in the morning or before bed. Volume is rarely addressed in the context we are referencing it here. Breath holds are not regularly prescribed or taught in a progressive and sustainable way. The predominant focus has been to slow breath rate, with particular attention given to extending the exhalation.

In the short term, extended exhales can indeed release stress, because exhalation is tied to the parasympathetic nervous system. This is the part of the ANS associated with the relaxation response. Extended exhales can take the edge off in moments of stress and, if utilized well, offer temporary relief. However, what is the impact on our physiology when we become reliant on extended exhales to cope with life's challenges? How does this habit alter our chemistry, our pH, and our health?

A person who consistently over-breathes may exhibit audible and frequent exhalations in the form of sighs, yawns, coughs, snores, and gasps. Teachers, receptionists, and salespeople face an occupational hazard of over-breathing simply by talking all day. Regardless of the impetus, once the big breathing pattern becomes established, it takes on a life of its own. Remember, the medulla responds to function: how we breathe habitually. Over-breathing can result in anxiety, exhaustion, overwhelm, and systemic inflammation. These symptoms often propel a feeling of urgency to breathe even more. As CO_2 levels drop, this vicious cycle accelerates—which explains why changing our breath habit requires an all-day and all-night retraining program and lots of svādhyāya and support.

As a yoga teacher or yoga therapist, it is critical that you have a good understanding of these basic respiratory principles. Otherwise you may mistakenly address the symptoms of breathlessness and stress in your students by suggesting they breathe *more*, thus exacerbating the situation.

The Power of CO_2

To emphasize how critical CO_2 is to our system, here are a few of the important processes that CO_2 governs in our body:

- increasing oxygenation of the tissue through the Bohr effect
- regulating pH
- dilating (expanding) smooth muscle, which is embedded in the airways, arteries, and in all the major organs (see Figures 3.7 and 3.8)

- reducing oxidative stress, decreasing inflammation (CO_2 is our body's best antioxidant!)
- having a sedative (quieting) effect on the nervous system.

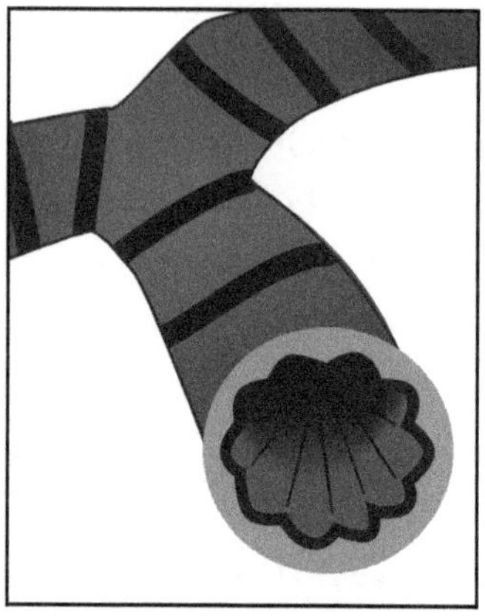

Figure 3.7 Normal Bronchiole Wrapped in Smooth Muscle

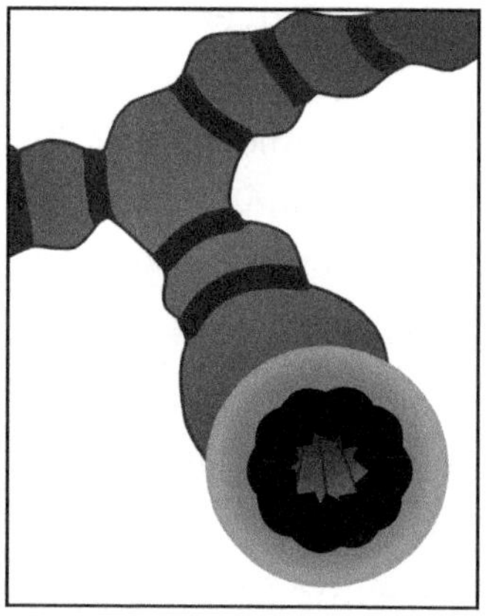

Figure 3.8 Asthmatic Bronchiole with Smooth Muscle Constricted Due to Low CO_2

It's important to note that CO_2 in its raw state is quite toxic, but within our body it dissociates. This means it changes its chemistry to become available to act as an acid/alkaline buffer and maintain pH in its healthy range.

As you become a more sophisticated observer of your breath rate and volume, there are a few biomechanical guidelines that will support your progression towards functional breathing. The first is to train yourself to breathe through your nose throughout the day, both on inhale and exhale. (If your nose is chronically stuffed, see the nose clearing practice described in Chapter 5 (Practice 5.1). The second is to develop an abdominal-diaphragmatic breathing pattern. With abdominal-diaphragmatic breathing, the chest remains passive during rest and with light exertion, such as simple daily tasks. The diaphragm and upper abdominals are the primary muscles that activate the base of the rib cage and pump the lower lobes of the lungs. Abdominal-diaphragmatic breathing supports the most efficient blood–gas exchange. These muscles can be strengthened and stretched like any other muscle through proper training. The embodied practices in Chapters 5–7 detail the means to develop healthy biomechanics. This topic will be thoroughly addressed there.

Additionally, as yoga teachers and therapists you'll need to learn how to cue for functional breathing in your classes by reminding students to breathe through the nose; abdominal-diaphragmatically; low, slow, and *silent*, while keeping the chest muscles passive (see Figure 3.9). Emphasize the importance of implementing this breath pattern throughout life, not just on the yoga mat.

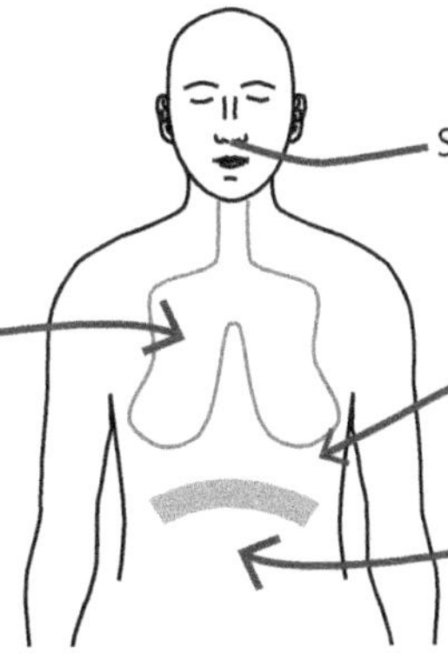

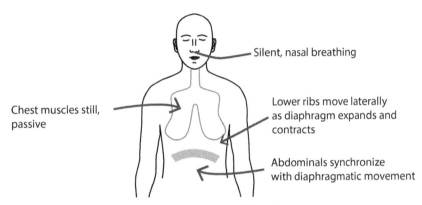

Figure 3.9 Functional Breathing

PRACTICE 3.1: MEASURING YOUR CO_2

It is not possible for a layperson to scientifically measure CO_2 levels without the aid of a fairly expensive device called a capnometer. These are used primarily by respiratory therapists or experts in the field of respiratory rehab and pulmonology. However, there is a simple, relatively accurate test even a layperson can use that is believed to be an indirect measurement of CO_2. This is known as the Comfortable Pause, or Control Pause, abbreviated as CP.[3] This simple test approximates one's comfort level with breath suspension or holding the breath after exhale. A higher CP is indicative of one's ability to tolerate higher levels of CO_2 and would depict a normal, healthy everyday breathing pattern. The inability to comfortably hold the breath after exhale may be indicative of low CO_2, marked by a constant call from the body to breathe more. This is one of the hallmarks of chronic hyperventilation—or an instilled pattern of breathing too much.

To take your Comfortable Pause (CP), all that is necessary is a stopwatch or a means to track seconds. The CP is always taken *after the exhale*.

The quintessential component for taking an accurate CP reading is reflected by the term *comfort*. The challenge for most people arises with the ego's attempt to want to push beyond the comfortable range to achieve a higher number. If you tend to strive for perfection, the practice itself will be a useful svādhyāya mirror. High achievers need to bring a sense of humor to this practice, to balance out their ambitious nature. Otherwise they'll find themselves frustrated. Pushing the breath will cause the CP to drop. When the pause is truly comfortable, the breath immediately following the pause will be calm and relaxed, as if there had been no breath suspension at all. If the breaths that follow the taking of the CP are at all labored or larger than the breaths before, that is an indication that the hold was pushed. I usually suggest shaving off a second or two in these cases, to stay honest with yourself. After all, the intention of taking your CP is to give you an accurate assessment of your breathing saṃskāra and CO_2 levels.

Taking Your CP

1. Sit quietly without speaking for 5 minutes and let your breath settle into its natural rhythm and flow.
2. Take a gentle inhale through your nose.
3. Exhale lightly out through your nose.
4. Pinch your nose and start the stopwatch.
5. Suspend your breath until you feel the first desire to breathe.
6. Release and look at the time.
7. That number reflects your CP.

Understanding Your CP

- A CP below 12 is an indication of very low CO_2 levels and will likely correlate with symptoms of hyperventilation syndrome (HVS). Symptoms of HVS can vary; a long list of them can be found in Chapter 4.
- A CP between 12 and 20 indicates low CO_2, with a vulnerable system easily triggered into reactivity.
- A CP consistently ranging between 20 and 25 indicates a more stable and resilient system.
- A CP between 30 and 40 correlates well to a "full tank" of CO_2, and will likely match someone with consistent vīrya (vitality) and good health.

Other Variables

If you take your CP after you've been very active or have been speaking a lot, the number will be affected by this. If you've had a cold and have been coughing or contending with allergies, this will also impact your CP. Alcohol and other foods will cause the CP to drop, as will time of day. This practice is intended to develop your familiarity with taking your CP and using it as a reflective tool for your life and EBA.

If you are in the below-20–25 range, train yourself to become a 24/7 functional breather. This is a great place to start. To reiterate, functional breathing at rest follows these parameters:

- nose breathing day and night
- abdominal-diaphragmatic breathing with little to no chest/accessory muscle involvement at rest
- light, silent, and steady breath, maintained at low volume.

If you are a yoga teacher, it is also important to become conscious of how you are cueing for the breath in your classes. Even if your own CP is well within the healthy range, consider how many of your students may be low-level hyperventilators. If you've been teaching big, audible ujjayi breathing, I'd suggest you shift to teaching functional breathing as your baseline. This is a safer way to go with breath practices in a group context, moving in the direction of "low and slow"—that is, low volume, low in the body (abdominal-diaphragmatic), and slow. (See the instructions for Subtle Breathing in Practice 4.1.)

PRACTICE 3.2: THE BREATH LOG

Use the following chart to help you monitor your CP three to four times a day for the next two weeks. Track how it changes from morning to night, at times of stress, and times of ease. Notice which activities seem to raise or lower it significantly. Begin to take your CP prior to your prāṇāyāma practices and then again at the end and notice if there is any notable change to your CP. Learn to observe and witness, conjuring equanimity and curiosity, rather than striving for change.

EXAMPLE

Comfortable Pause Tracking Chart

Date	*Time*	*CP*	*Comments/Reflections*
6/25	*8 a.m.*	*12 sec.*	*I had a restless night's sleep. The room was too hot and my back was hurting. I had to pee 3x, so am moving super slow today. Feeling very stiff and achy.*
6/25	*12 p.m.*	*15 sec.*	*I forced myself to go to yoga class and I felt better afterwards. When I sat in the car and took my CP, I was surprised it was higher than in the morning.*
6/25	*4 p.m.*	*11 sec.*	*Late afternoons are always hard as I often have a big energy drop. Sometimes I have coffee or sugar (I love cookies) to give me a boost. I decided to take my CP after I downed my latte and snickerdoodle. I wasn't surprised that it had dropped. I wonder if it's the time of day or the food??*

CP = Comfortable Pause

Comfortable Pause Tracking Chart

Date	Time	CP	Comments/Reflections

CP = Comfortable Pause

Comfortable Pause Tracking Chart

Date	Time	CP	Comments/Reflections

CP = Comfortable Pause

Comfortable Pause Tracking Chart

Date	Time	CP	Comments/Reflections

CP = Comfortable Pause

Comfortable Pause Tracking Chart

Date	Time	CP	Comments/Reflections

CP = Comfortable Pause

4

SUBTLE BREATHING, THE FOUNDATION OF FUNCTION

The definition of hyperventilation is breathing in excess of metabolic production of CO_2, resulting in blood CO_2 levels dropping below normal (normal = 40 mmHg). Hyperventilation syndrome (HVS) is often missed by routine medical examinations, yet approximately 9.5 percent of the population have been found to present with HVS.[1] Children who hyperventilate often exhibit symptoms such as asthma, behavior problems, sleep disturbance, and chronic respiratory infections.[2] Both stress and pain increase respiratory rate and, when chronic, can instigate hyperventilation.

On average, a healthy person breathes 15,000–20,000 times a day. People with chronic pain, illness, or anxiety, and those who talk for a living often breathe two to three times more than normal (both faster and more volume) (see Figure 4.1).[3]

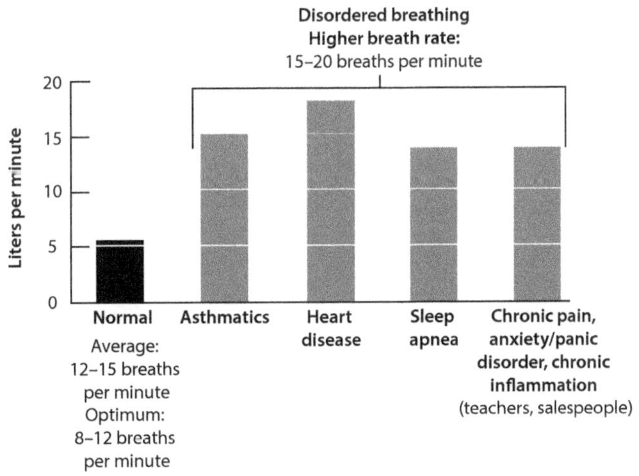

Figure 4.1 Breath Volume and Rate Comparison Chart

Many yoga students and yoga therapy clients seek out yoga specifically to help them manage stress or chronic pain. They often describe common maladies which symptomatically may be associated with hyperventilation. Unfortunately, many breathing techniques currently taught in contemporary yoga classes emphasize taking big, audible breaths, often rapidly. Over time, this can exacerbate HVS and may subsequently result in a subtle increase in symptoms over time, while simultaneously creating a short-term sense of relaxation or calm.

HVS SYMPTOMS[4]

- shortness of breath
- chest breathing
- anxiety/panic
- asthma, chronic obstructive pulmonary disease (COPD)
- insomnia
- snoring/sleep apnea
- restless leg syndrome
- anaphylactic reactions
- temporomandibular joint disorder (TMJD)
- chronic cough
- stuffy nose, sinusitis, hay fever
- anterior head carriage
- postural issues
- heartburn/gastroesophageal reflux disease (GERD)
- migraines
- muscle cramps
- multiple chemical sensitivities
- muscle pain
- myofascial pain
- mood swings
- poor exercise tolerance
- poor immunity
- poor memory
- swollen lymph glands
- dry skin, mouth, eyes
- high blood pressure
- low blood pressure
- food allergies
- constipation
- bloating
- excessive flatulence
- brain fatigue
- abdominal spasms
- anal irritation
- hemorrhoids
- food cravings
- sluggishness
- depression
- chronic fatigue
- osteoporosis
- seizure disorder
- dizziness
- cold hands/feet, Raynaud's syndrome
- recurrent bladder infections
- recurrent vaginal infections
- recurrent skin rashes

The Challenge of Changing the Breath Saṃskāra

Breathing is a difficult saṃskāra to change, because our habit of breathing is pervasive and mostly unconscious. As the yogis pointed out, we can only change patterns that are conscious. The breath pattern is particularly tricky to shift because, as mentioned in the previous chapter, CO_2 levels are closely tied to pH. Chronic hyperventilation changes the set point of the medulla, leading to sustained low levels of CO_2. Once HVS is set in place, sympathetic arousal of the autonomic nervous system is easily triggered, perpetuating higher volume and erratic respiratory rates (see Figure 4.2).

This will further destabilize pH, making the body less able to process acid, and ultimately less tolerant of CO_2. This condition is called respiratory alkalosis. Many of the symptoms related to HVS correspond to this imbalance in pH. For instance, people with HVS are more prone to chronic inflammatory conditions like irritable bowel syndrome (IBS) and gastroesophageal reflux disease (GERD). Frequent urination, especially at night, can also be symptomatic of HVS. Over-breathing during the day has been correlated with snoring and sleep apnea. Low-level hyperventilators may exhibit reduced exercise tolerance, tire quickly, or remain very sore after exertion due to high levels of unbuffered lactic acid in their blood. Additionally, breathing hard and fast consumes large quantities of oxygen in order to recruit the accessory breathing muscles of the chest.[5]

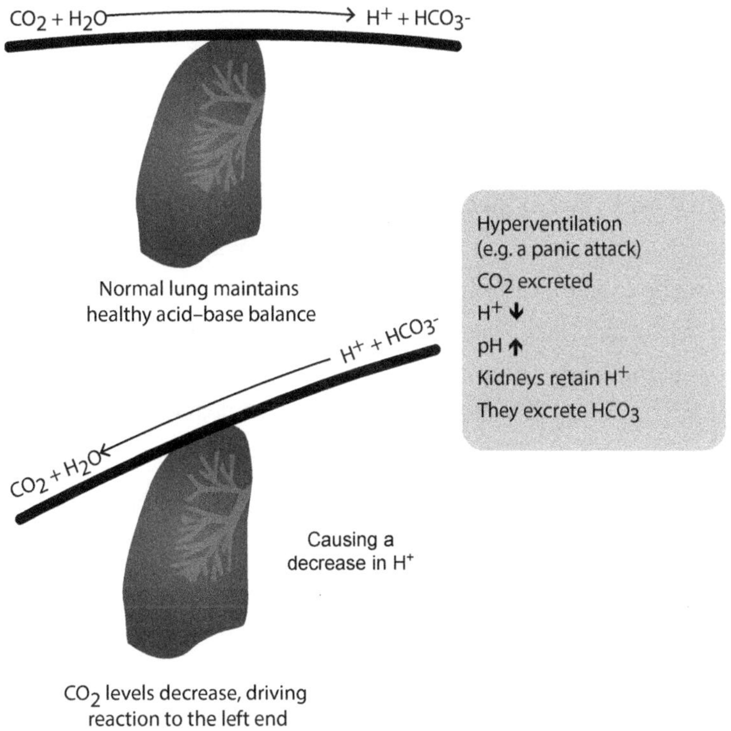

Figure 4.2 Respiratory Alkalosis

The challenge in the retraining process is that the medulla doesn't reset easily—the longer the pattern of hyperventilation has been set in place, the more arduous it is to change it. Taking a big sigh or gasp will alleviate the immediate sense of breathlessness, but it perpetuates the chemical imbalance that promotes hyperventilation. Chronic hyperventilation is associated with the following disordered breathing patterns: mouth, chest, paradoxical (reversed), and belly breathing. Subtle Breathing (described below) explores a reduced breathing practice designed to gradually (over the course of weeks and months) elevate CO_2 tolerance and recalibrate the set point of the medulla, making the breath functional. Functional breathing supports vitality, health, and the filling of your prāṇic reservoir. Each practice provides a direct deposit into your Energy Bank Account (EBA). For this reason, the Subtle Breath will form the basis for all Restore Your Prāṇa practices.

The consequence of long-term hyperventilation is that while the body suffers from poor oxygenation, the accompanying feeling of breathlessness creates a strong aversion to breathing less. Subtle Breathing is based on the Buteyko Method of Reduced Breathing, as well as the description of Akasha Breathing from the yoga lineage.[6]

PRACTICE 4.1: SUBTLE BREATHING

Learning to make the breath subtle by reducing rate and volume is a challenging task. The practice of Subtle Breathing several times a day in 10–15-minute intervals will affect your autonomic nervous system and your blood chemistry, especially if you tend to be an over-breather. Sprinkling the Subtle Breathing practice throughout the day maintains a level of svādhyāya, which can help you draw connections between your breathing saṃskāra and the state of your mind and body. This consistent reinforcement makes it easier to keep the breath slow and low, and illuminates the times you fall back into your habitual patterns.

The practice of Subtle Breathing will assist you in the management of your EBA. View your dietary, speech, exercise, and sleep habits not as separate events, but rather as part of the larger prāṇavayu picture. Begin to piece together cause-and-effect correlations between your breath patterns and your physiological functions. In this way, pin the prāṇamaya to the forefront of your mind. Every choice symbolizes either a move towards greater function or a solidifying of the old pattern of imbalance. In essence, restraining and retraining the breath requires nothing short of constant vigilance. This is why prāṇāyāma is considered the greatest tapas practice of all!

At this point in your svādhyāya process, you probably have a good sense of your daily breath patterns and your average CP. While you may not identify yourself as being a chronic hyperventilator—remember, only approximately 10 per cent of the population have measurably low levels of CO_2—I would still recommend working with the Subtle Breathing practice to experience how it feels to refine the breath to a state of sūkṣma, or subtlety.

Subtle Breathing can be practiced seated upright in a chair, or on a cushion on the floor (Photos 1, 2, 3). Choose whichever position is most comfortable and relaxing for you. If the seated position is accompanied by pain or discomfort, it is best to work semi-reclined, or even supine with ample support under the neck and knees (Photo 4). This will relax the spinal musculature and facilitate undistracted focus on the breath.

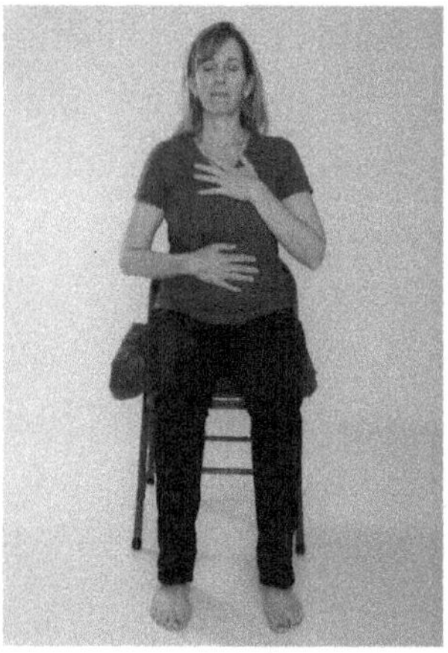

Photo 1 Subtle Breathing on Chair with Hi-Low Hand Position

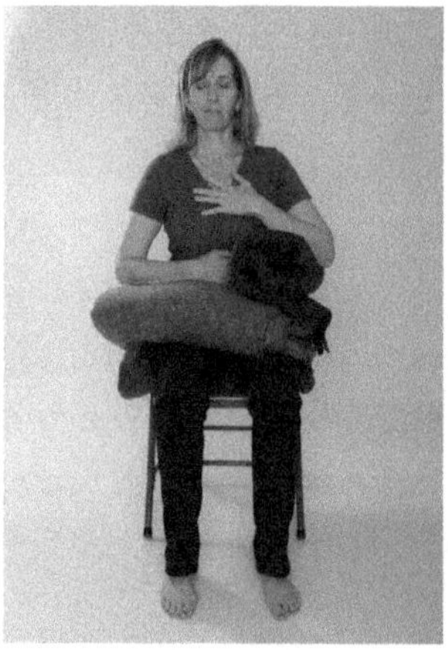

Photo 2 Subtle Breathing with Prop Support

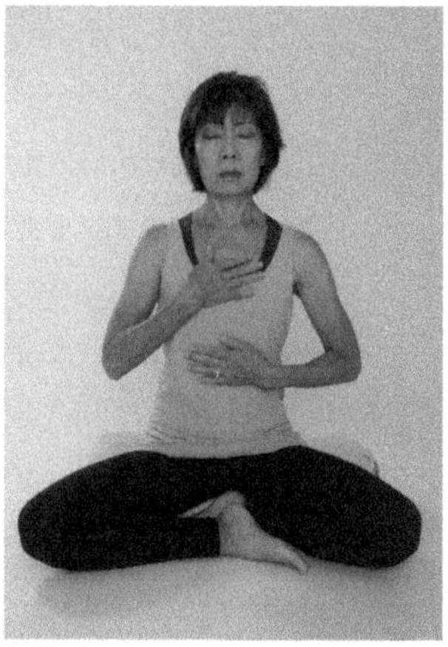

Photo 3 Subtle Breathing Sitting on Floor

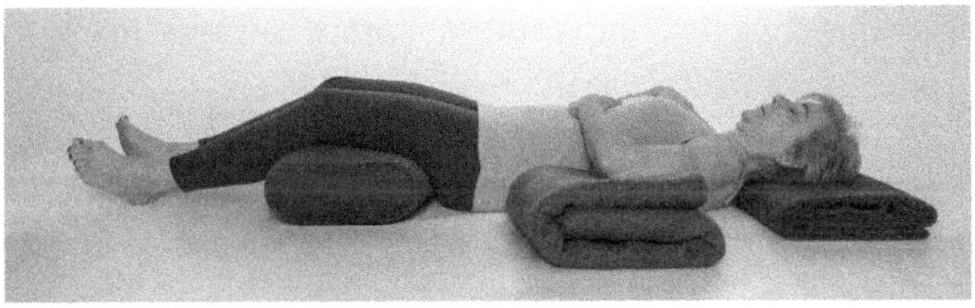

Photo 4 Supine Breathing with Support under Neck and Knees, Hands in Hi-Low Position—Arms Propped

More about the Subtle Breath

It is valuable to acknowledge at the outset that it is *much* easier (and more comfortable) for most people to breathe more than it is to breathe less. Breathing less is like portion control; it's a kind of air diet. As with caloric intake, we can become accustomed to higher quantities of substances than our body can process well. This applies to air much as it does to sugar and carbs. With habituation, the excessive volume becomes equated in our mind with the feeling of satiation. Even though reducing the load is healthier for us, it can sometimes feel as if we're starving. Therefore, it is important to work with the subtle, reduced breath slowly and consistently. We need to reinforce our intention to change the way the brain is calling for breath. To make the change lasting and the practice sustainable, we also need to read our levels of tolerance accurately and not try to force or push the breath in a way that causes stress. The Subtle Breath requires a high degree of introspection and attention.

If you feel sleepy or drowsy during practice, it is likely that you were not riding the edge of air hunger but rather stayed in your comfort zone. Gaining the benefit of Subtle Breathing requires dropping below the level of pure comfort to another state, one in which every breath requires attention and fine-tuning. Much like riding a surf board, you need to observe every wave and adjust your balance to stay afloat. You want to learn to calibrate as you practice, in order to keep yourself in what I refer to as the *zen-zone of tolerable discomfort.*

PRACTICE 4.2: SUBTLE BREATHING—FULL PRACTICE

Recommended practice: 4–6 times a day (for 3–5 minutes per session).

To gain the most svādhyāya from this practice, I recommend you take your CP before starting, and also again at the end. If you have a CP below 10 or any kind of cardiovascular condition, please build the practice slowly. Resist the urge to push, as this could elevate your heart rate or bring on feelings of anxiety. Even if your CP is higher than 10, you'll discover that pushing beyond your tolerance will likely result in you taking a large gasp of air reflexively, defeating the intention of the practice.

1. Sit in a Seated Mountain Pose with your spine erect (Photos 1 and 3).
2. Begin by taking your CP and make note of it. (Find instructions for taking your CP in Chapter 3.)

3. Place one hand on your chest, and your other hand just below the front of your rib cage, in the area of your solar plexus.
4. If your arm position is uncomfortable, use pillows or towels to prop your arms, so your neck and shoulders can relax fully (Photo 2).
5. Breathe softly through your nose.
6. Pacify the muscles of your chest. Quiet any movement in your upper rib cage. Relax tension in your neck.
7. Keep your lips together throughout the practice, for inhalation and exhalation.
8. Emphasize a soft lateral flare of your lower ribs with the inhale, and a gentle inward contraction with the exhale.
9. Place attention on the feeling of your breath as it passes through your nostrils.
10. Progressively lighten the movement of your breath as if making the breath "invisible."
11. As you breathe in, visualize the Subtle Breath permeating every cell within you, as if you are breathing in space rather than air.
12. Consistently lighten the exhale so it becomes thread-like, imperceptible.
13. Throughout, maintain a silent breath with all movement becoming less discernible with each cycle.
14. Discover the soft edge of air hunger, where you are not "starving," yet are aware of a desire to take in more.
15. Maintain a sustainable level of "hunger" without pushing yourself into the need to gasp for a breath for another 3–5 minutes.

Note: If you slow the breath beyond what is sustainable, the volume will increase. If you lower the volume too much, the rate will pick up. Find the *tolerable* level of low and slow breathing and maintain that for the duration of the practice. (Use a timer or stopwatch.)

16. As you come out of the practice, release your hands and relax your breath.
17. Continue to breathe gently through your nose.
18. Notice the contrast between your normal breath rate and volume and the effect of Subtle Breathing on your system.
19. Continue to breathe naturally for 1–2 minutes, allowing your breath to settle.
20. Repeat another round of Subtle Breathing, building to 3–4 minutes as is tolerable.
21. Rest again and observe.
22. If possible, do another round, building to 4–5 minutes.

23. Eventually build your tolerance to sustain your Subtle Breathing time to 5–10 minutes per round (take a 1–2 minute resting-breath break between rounds as necessary).

24. End the practice with a period of natural breathing for 2–3 minutes.

25. Take your CP again.

26. Track this information on the Subtle Breathing Chart below.

Note: The lower your CP at the start, the more quickly you will experience sensations of breathlessness. Work gently, always maintaining a quality of relaxation even while experiencing the challenge of breathing less. You may experience a variety of sensations that are unusual as you practice. These are quite normal and may include:

- sensations of warmth in the limbs or center of your body
- sensations of cold in the limbs or center of your body
- an increase of saliva in your mouth
- a sense of moistening in your eyes or slightly glazed/diffused gaze
- a clearing of your nose—especially if there was congestion prior to practice
- an opening of your sinus passageways
- a feeling of calm, alert awareness in your mind
- relaxation in your body without sleepiness.

It is helpful to monitor your heart rate (HR) by taking your pulse at your wrist or at your throat before and after practice as another means of self-regulation. This will also give you an opportunity to gain insight into how the practice is serving you. I recommend taking your HR after your CP. At the end of a good Subtle Breathing practice, your CP will increase by a few seconds and your HR will decrease or remain unchanged. A CP that is lower and HR that is higher indicates that you pushed beyond your capacity. Please note that daily fluctuations in both CP and HR are normal within 1–4 seconds/beats. This process is non-linear. That is to say, your breath pattern is reflective of your lifestyle, inclusive of the whole prāṇamaya in addition to the usual vṛttis, such as thoughts and feelings: sleep patterns, dietary habits, exercise routines, and emotional states. All of these will affect the numbers and the felt sense during the practice. The Subtle Breathing Tracking Chart will help you see patterns of connection between your breath and your life more clearly.

EXAMPLE

Subtle Breathing Tracking Chart

Date	*Time of day*	*CP before/ after*	*HR before/ after*	*SB*	*Comments/Reflections*
7/12/19	*7 a.m.*	*16/ 18*	*72/72*	*3 min.* *rest* *4 min.* *rest*	*I still find it really hard to settle into the SB with the first round. My chest feels tight and I have to fight the desire to take a big breath. The second round is easier and I do feel some warming of my hands (which is great because they're always cold!) and more saliva in my mouth. By the end of the practice I feel more relaxed. I especially notice less tension in my neck and jaw. My mind feels quieter too.*
7/12/19	*3 p.m.*	*15/19*	*72/68*	*4 min.* *rest* *5 min.*	*The morning was super hectic and I had lunch with friends, so was gabbing a lot. Then my daughter called and she's having a hard time, so I ended up talking to her for nearly an hour. I had to take a nap after that, I was so drained. I felt better when I woke up and took the dog for a 30 min. walk, which was refreshing. Read a little bit and then remembered to do my practice. At first my CP was lower than in the morning and felt a little pushed (maybe it should've been 14), but I was able to settle into the Subtle Breath more quickly and it felt very relaxing. I don't think I've felt it quite like that before. My ending CP was quite a bit higher than when I started and my HR lower. I was happy about that. Felt a bit more energy than usual through the evening.*

CP = Comfortable Pause (note before/after); HR = heart rate (note before/after);
SB = Subtle Breath (length of time of practice, e.g. 4 minutes)

Subtle Breathing Tracking Chart

Date	Time of day	CP before/after	HR before/after	SB	Comments/Reflections

CP = Comfortable Pause (note before/after); HR = heart rate (note before/after); SB = Subtle Breath (length of time of practice, e.g. 4 minutes)

Subtle Breathing Tracking Chart

Date	Time of day	CP before/after	HR before/after	SB	Comments/Reflections

CP = Comfortable Pause (note before/after); HR = heart rate (note before/after); SB = Subtle Breath (length of time of practice, e.g. 4 minutes)

Subtle Breathing Tracking Chart

Date	Time of day	CP before/after	HR before/after	SB	Comments/Reflections

CP = Comfortable Pause (note before/after); HR = heart rate (note before/after); SB = Subtle Breath (length of time of practice, e.g. 4 minutes)

Subtle Breathing Tracking Chart

Date	Time of day	CP before/after	HR before/after	SB	Comments/Reflections

CP = Comfortable Pause (note before/after); HR = heart rate (note before/after); SB = Subtle Breath (length of time of practice, e.g. 4 minutes)

Additional resources

Patrick McKeown, author of *The Oxygen Advantage*, offers a downloadable reduced breathing app that has served many of my students well as they are learning this practice. With his lovely Irish accent, this app is like a yoga nidra (a particular type of guided meditation), and provides a fabulous way to begin the day, or to help you reduce the breath to prepare for sleep. It is available through the iTunes app store: ButeykoClinicInternational Self Help Program.

5 THE NOSE VERSUS THE MOUTH

We'll begin our exploration into the biomechanics of breathing by examining the importance of nasal breathing and problems associated with chronic mouth breathing, particularly in children. The practices in this chapter work primarily with the tongue and jaw, and can easily be added into your daily routine. Dysfunctional speech patterns can contribute to over-breathing and hyperventilation, and the practices in this chapter are intended to help you transform those saṃskāras as well.

The All-Important Nose

It may seem obvious, but the nose was designed for breathing. Surprisingly, many people bypass the nose and breathe through their mouth. The importance of nose breathing cannot be overstated as the nose provides the first line of defense for our immune system. Among its many other functions, the nose warms, humidifies, and cleans the air we breathe, preparing it for the lungs. The nasal cavity controls airflow through the upper airways (see Figure 5.1). Nose breathing is linked to both the autonomic nervous system and movement of our most important breathing muscle, the respiratory diaphragm. Our limbic brain (the emotional center) and our sense of smell are connected to our sense of survival. Nasal breathing supports oxygen uptake and good perfusion of O_2 and CO_2 in the lungs.

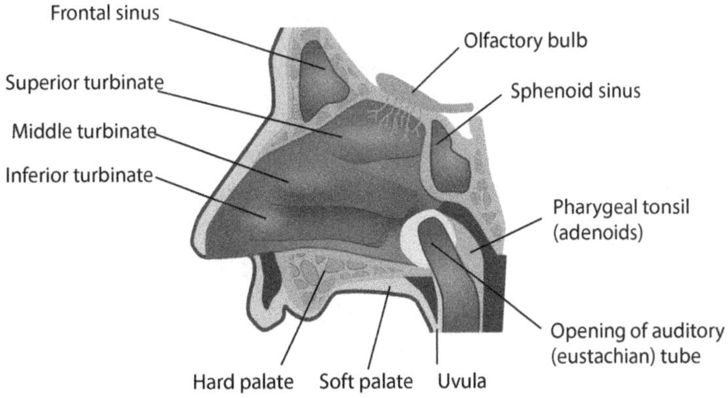

Figure 5.1 The Nasal Cavity

Mouth and chest breathing often develop together. Both are linked to sympathetic activation of the nervous system, which in turn can increase anxiety and nasal congestion. Mouth breathing has been associated with cognitive impairment such as memory and concentration difficulties, as well as headaches. Conditions like TMJD, anterior head carriage (forward head position), and chronic neck and shoulder tension often develop as a result of consistent mouth breathing. Additionally, mouth breathing contributes to high rates of dental cavities, gum disease, and bad breath. It has also been implicated in sleep issues, such as insomnia and apnea. Mouth breathing can be the result of structural obstructions such as a severe deviated septum, or, in the case of children, chronically inflamed adenoids or tonsils (see Figure 5.2). However, most of the time mouth breathing is simply a matter of habit. Apparently, the less we use our nose, the stuffier it will become, which reinforces the need to breathe through the mouth. Over time, this can result in upper airway constriction and reduces diaphragmatic recruitment by half.

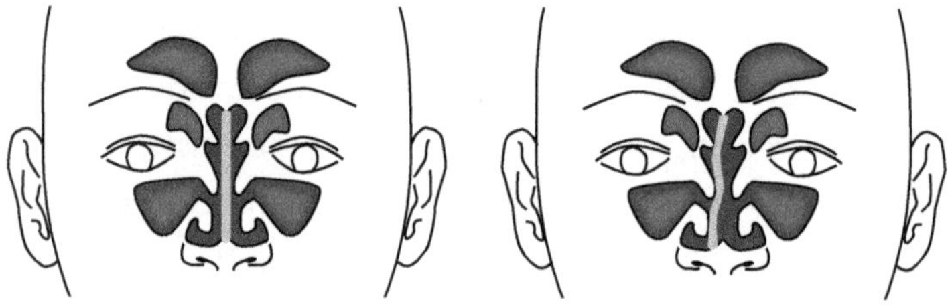

Figure 5.2 Normal and Deviated Septum

Dr. Buteyko theorized that with chronic hyperventilation, the body produces mucus as a defense mechanism for excessive loss of CO_2.[1] From an Ayurvedic perspective, this idea makes sense. Ayurvedically, over-breathing would be considered a derangement of vata dośa. With the incessant movement of the breath at high volumes, chafing of the airways occurs. The lining becomes irritated and inflamed (pitta dośa), much like our hands and lips do when they are exposed to cold, dry wind. The ensuing inflammatory response activates kapha, which lays down a protective coating of mucus, similar to an application of lotion or balm we'd apply to soothe chapped skin. The combination of the swelling and narrowing of the "wind-tunnel" will in essence impede the flow of air. If we address this doshic imbalance by simply clearing out the mucus through the use of antihistamines or even a neti pot, we will experience only short-term relief. As long as the breath continues to "blow" excessively, it is as if we're running a hurricane through our system. If, instead, we train ourselves to breathe less, more lightly, and through the nose, we'll achieve greater success because we'll be addressing the source of the problem by reducing vata. This in turn will calm the irritation and stem the over-production of mucus. (See Figure 5.3.)

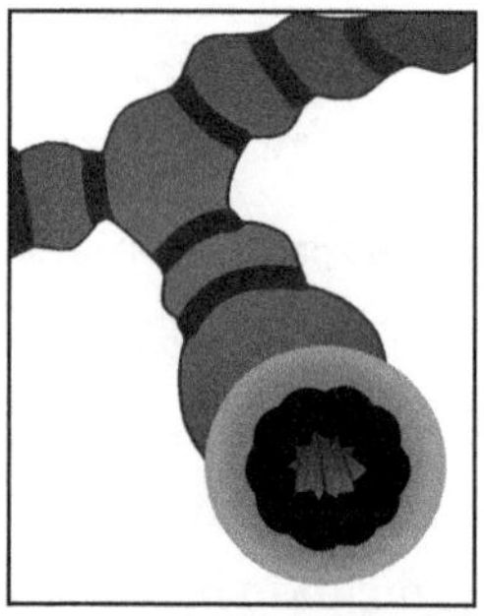

Figure 5.3 An Ayurvedic Perspective: Irritated Airway Due to Over-Breathing—Build-Up of Inflammation (Pitta) and Mucus (Kapha)

Mouth breathing in children has become a pervasive issue and can affect facial and jaw development, sleep, and behavior (see Figure 5.4). If not addressed early in life, mouth breathing can have serious health ramifications as these children reach adolescence and move into adulthood.[2] Functional orthodontists and myofunctional therapists can assist children who are mouth-breathers in becoming nose-breathers. Yoga teachers who work with children have a particular responsibility to teach parents about the importance of functional breathing and to teach children to breathe correctly in their yoga classes.

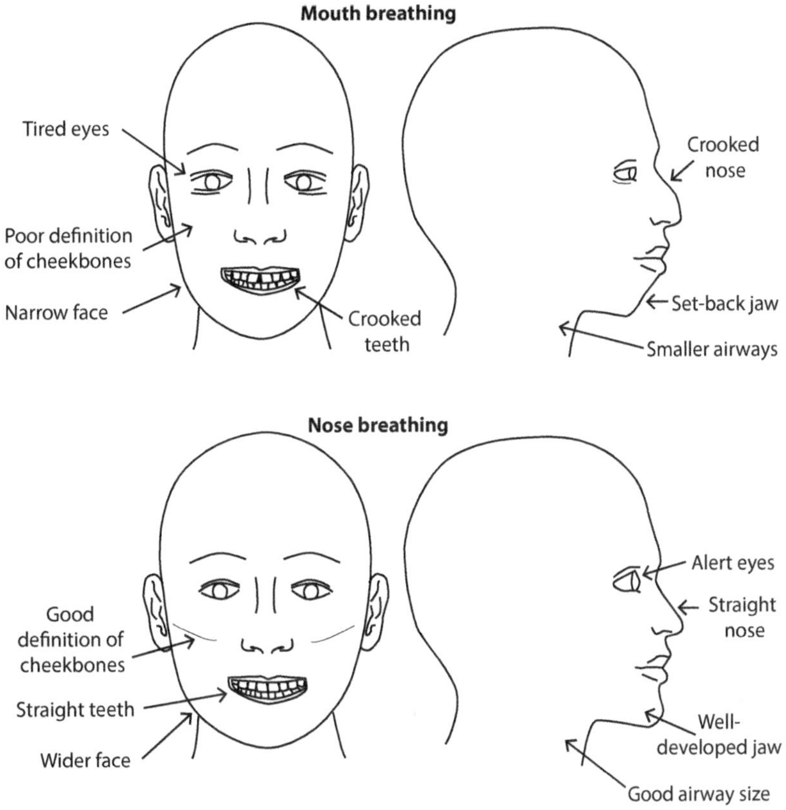

Figure 5.4 Facial Development with Mouth versus Nose Breathing

Minding the Tongue and Proper Speech

The tongue is a particularly strong and important muscle that rarely gets much attention. Correct placement of the tongue requires it to stay pressed firmly to the upper palate. Mouth-breathers tend to have flaccid tongues that rest to the bottom of the mouth. While this may seem insignificant, as far back as the Vedic teachings tongue mūdras were considered an extension of prāṇāyāma practice. Modern experts in breath retraining also consider exercises that condition and stretch the tongue critical in transforming the mouth-breathing pattern. Jiva Mūdra reinforces the seal of the lips and maintains space in the jaw. It is an excellent every-day, all-day svādhyāya practice for any mouth-breather!

It's one thing to develop the nose-breathing habit when we have no need to open the mouth. However, learning to breathe correctly during speech can be a challenge. For people whose vocation requires constant talking, learning to breathe in a functional manner while speaking is a worthwhile endeavor. This includes becoming aware of the tendency to gasp and breathe heavily through the mouth in between words or phrases. Learning to pause and inhale through the nose during conversational speech is a significant aspect of breath retraining that can make a qualitative difference in the level of fatigue you feel at the end of the day.

As yoga teachers, we can train ourselves to identify dysfunctional mouth- and chest-breathing patterns in our students. Through education and reinforcement of functional biomechanics during our yoga classes, we can support our students in transforming their breath saṃskāras and improving their health. The following simple practices can easily be woven into your daily routine, your personal practice, or, if you are teaching, into your yoga classes. They will increase your svādhyāya and support the development of more functional breathing patterns in life.

Practices for Exploration and Transformation

PRACTICE 5.1: NOSE CLEARING (PHOTOS 5 AND 6)

This practice is useful when your nose is stuffy due to colds, hay fever, allergies, or chronic congestion. It can be done intermittently throughout the day to your level of comfort. Keep your lips closed throughout the process.

1. Take a gentle breath in and a gentle breath out through your nose.
2. After the exhale, pinch your nose and hold, maintaining a tight seal.
3. Rock your head side to side or up and down—move gently to avoid any kind of discomfort or pull on your neck.
4. When you feel the need to breathe, stop the rocking, release the nose-pinch, and take a gentle breath in through your nose.
5. Pause. Feel. Repeat 4–6 times until your nasal passage feels more open.

This practice can be taught to young children as well as adults. It was my granddaughter's favorite. Every time she did it, her airways opened, making it easier for her to breathe. She experienced it as a kind of magic trick.

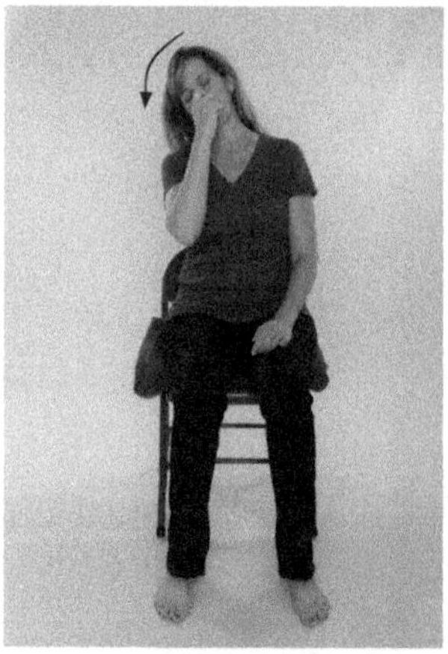

Photo 5

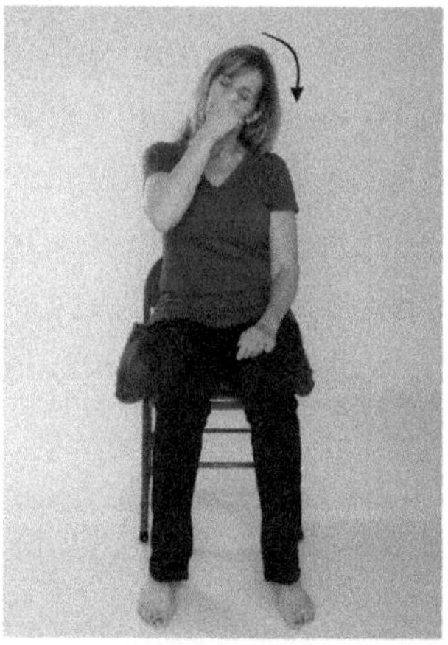

Photo 6

Use the space below to write a brief reflection of your experience with the nose-clearing practice. What did you observe? Did it relieve some of the congestion? On average, how many repetitions of the practice were needed to clear the nose? Was your response to the process always the same?

When the Nose-Clearing Practice Isn't Enough

If the nose-clearing practice doesn't seem to be working, try turning up your body's internal heat. Jogging in place or walking briskly up and down your hallway while holding your breath will increase CO_2 levels and help open your airways. Never hold your nose to the point where you find yourself gasping or having to open your mouth to breathe. After each short breath-hold, be sure to breathe in through your nose.

Sometimes, the nose is so plugged, more help is needed. A neti pot sinus wash can help tremendously with clearing out extra mucus from the sinus passageways. It is highly recommended that you use sterile saline for your neti pot to ensure safe use; tap water alone should never be used. Keep in mind that if over-breathing (vata derangement) is causing inflammation, mucus is the body's way of protecting the irritated airways and maintaining CO_2. Saline wash can cleanse, but can also strip the natural protective coating from your nasal cavity. It is important to follow up your neti pot washes with a light coat of olive or nasya (nasal) oil. Apply to the inside of your nose after you've used your neti. Banyan Botanicals has aromatic, organic nasya oil available at www.banyanbotanicals.com.

PRACTICE 5.2: SERIES TO DEVELOP THE TONGUE

Use the Developing the Tongue Chart below to track your experience of the following practices.

(A) Jiva Mūdra

A toned tongue can go far to alleviate jaw pain, reduce tension headaches, and facilitate nasal breathing. Jiva Mūdra, or the tongue lock, is a practice that supports proper placement of the tongue in the mouth. Imagine that you are saying the letter "N" silently, and feel the flat of your tongue parked up into your upper palate. Observe the space this creates in your jaw joint, preventing clenching and grinding. Employ this position of your tongue consistently throughout the day to help reduce mouth breathing and condition the muscles of your face. Hold this position as you are able during your āsana, prāṇāyāma, and meditation practices. If you are a mouth-breather, create specific times for remembering to do Jiva Mūdra during the day, such as every traffic light, when you use the bathroom, before you check your cell phone, while washing dishes. Eventually, with practice, you will develop the saṃskāra and your tongue will stay parked up top.

(B) Washing the Teeth with the Tongue (Photo 7)

1. Close your mouth.
2. Place your tongue on the far right side, pressing it into your upper teeth and gums.
3. Slowly wash your tongue across your upper teeth and gumline over to your left side.
4. Stretch your tongue to your left lower gumline and proceed to wash across to your right.
5. Circle right to left 5 times.
6. Reverse the direction and circle left to right.
7. Practice 2–3 times a day.

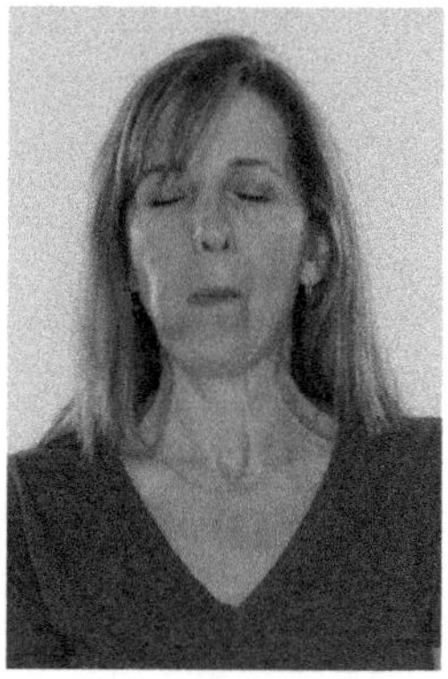

Photo 7

(C) Tongue Extensions (Photos 8 and 9)

This is a great one to bring out the kid in all of us. Who doesn't love sticking out their tongue—especially at the teacher!

1. Stick your tongue straight out as far as you can, holding it parallel like a plank for 10 seconds.
2. Stretch it out and as far to the right as you can and hold 10 seconds.
3. Stretch it out and as far to the left as you can and hold 10 seconds.
4. Try to touch your nose with your tongue and hold 10 seconds.
5. Try to touch your chin with your tongue and hold 10 seconds.

You may be surprised at how quickly your tongue fatigues. If 10 seconds feels too long, start with 5 and build up your endurance. Start with this series once a day and then build to twice a day.

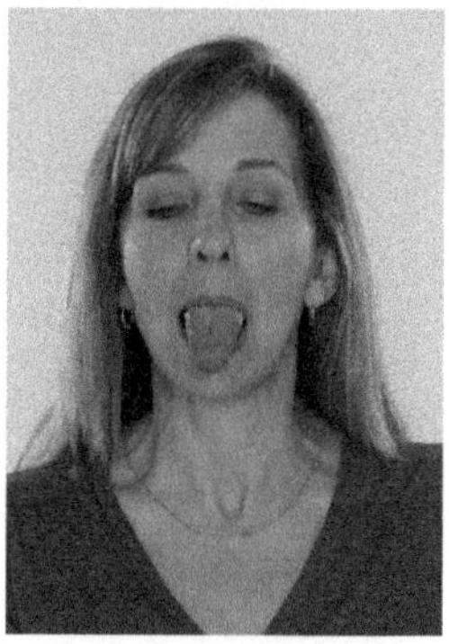

Photo 8

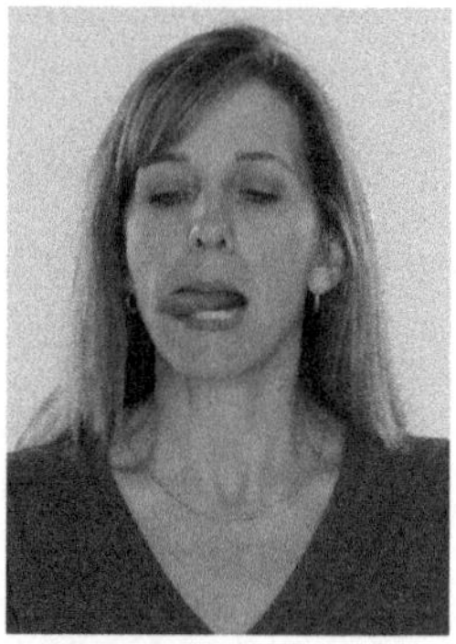

Photo 9

(D) Kechari Mūdra (Photos 10 and 11)

Kechari Mūdra is considered the king among mūdras. You could think of it as a "tongue lift," as it requires stretching the tongue up into the cavity of the soft palate. In its most extreme forms, the tongue was stretched to roll back to the uvula at the back of the throat. Kechari is mentioned in the Gheranda Samhita, and the Hatha Yoga Pradipika, and was touted as having remarkable healing capabilities. It was said to enable the practitioner to taste the amrit, or divine nectar that flows from the sinuses down into the back of the throat.

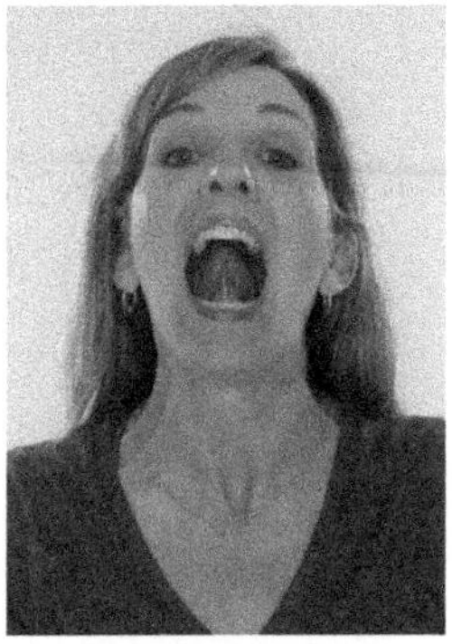

Photo 10

The form of kechari offered here is designed to support healthy tone of the tongue, and to increase awareness of how and where the tongue is placed in the mouth as it relates to breathing.

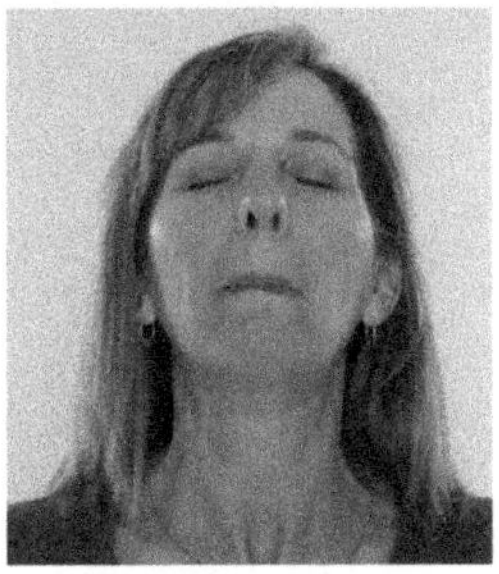

Photo 11

1. Sit comfortably.
2. With your mouth closed, extend your tongue up until it touches the back of your upper palate.
3. Reach back as far as you can to touch your soft palate.
4. If your frenum is short, it may take weeks or months to stretch it out.
5. As you are able, slip your tongue up into the cavity of your soft palate. Reach the tip up as high as you can and hold it there for 10 seconds.
6. Repeat 4–6 times or until fatigued.

Once you are able to perform Kechari Mūdra comfortably, build your endurance until you are able to sustain it for longer periods of time.

(E) Clucking with Mouth Closed

The Clucking exercise was shared by a couple of fabulous myofunctional therapists at the Buteyko Breathing Educators Conference some years ago and is to this day one of my favorite tongue exercises. The initial challenge of it took me by surprise and made me aware of how deconditioned my tongue actually was. Start with your mouth open and "cluck" by thrusting your tongue against the hard, upper palate. Make the sound crisp and clear. Now repeat the exercise with your mouth closed. Cluck until tired. Rest. Repeat. Have fun! Imagine clucking while holding Tree Pose or Warrior 3!

(F) Shītali/Shītkari—Tongue Breath (Photos 12 and 13)

These two variations on breathing use the tongue as a funnel, or as a valve to channel the inhalation. The moisture of the tongue helps to cool the breath and can help when the body is over-heated or to calm an agitated mind. They work much like a damp cloth in front of a fan helps to ventilate a stuffy room with a cool breeze. They may also be useful in bringing more awareness to the action of the tongue and placement in the mouth. That said, for those who tend to be mouth-breathers, I do not recommend these two as starting points for practice. It would be better to focus on developing nose breathing as your default pattern and return to these prāṇāyāmas once you've mastered that.

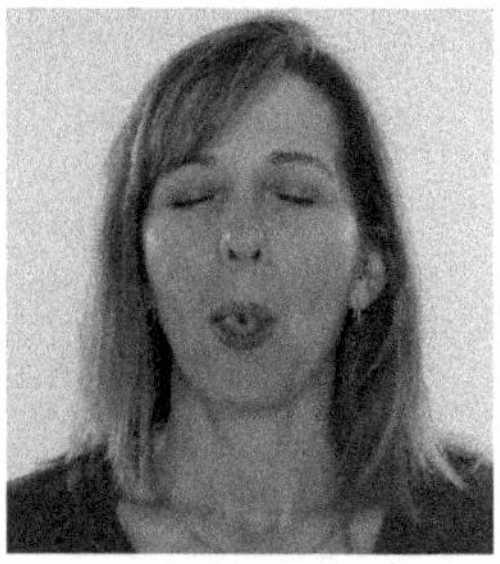

Photo 10

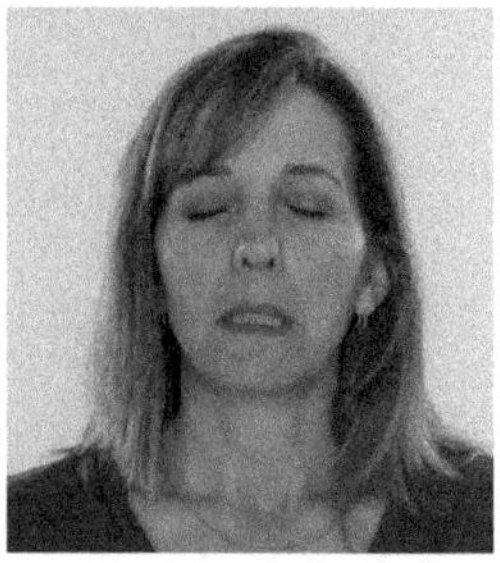

Photo 11

Shītali: If you are able to curl your tongue into a tube like a straw, draw the breath lightly in this way. At the end of the inhale, close your lips and curl your tongue back, so the bottom of the tongue presses into your upper palate. Holding this position, gently exhale through your nose.

Shītkari is an adaptation of this practice and is useful for those who are unable to perform the tongue curl. In this variation, you press the tip of your tongue into the back side of the top teeth at the gumline and gently suck in through slightly open lips. Exhalation is the same as with shītali.

Write a brief description of your experience with these practices each week over the next month.

EXAMPLE

Developing the Tongue Chart

Week 1

Type of Practice	*Frequency*	*Reflections on Practice*
Jiva Mūdra	*Try to maintain through the day*	*Felt awkward initially. Now, it's becoming easier. My jaw feels more relaxed as I practice. Still have to remind myself frequently to press up instead of letting the tongue slack to my lower palate.*
Washing the Teeth with the Tongue	*2–3x*	*This makes my jaw ache—I get super tired after just doing it 3–4x. I know it's good for me, but it's hard to make myself do it every day. I'm going to try to practice more in the next week.*
Tongue Extensions	*2–3x*	*Like the tongue washing, I'm amazed at how tired my tongue gets. Who knew it was so weak? Especially the straight forward extension. Super hard!*
Kechari Mūdra	*every day*	*I like this. I don't know why, but it feels really good to stretch my tongue up this way. It seems to relax my jaw and I feel like there's more space in my throat afterwards. I try to do Kechari Mūdra before I do my Subtle Breathing as a kind of preparation.*
Clucking with Mouth Closed	*1x*	*I only did this once and it felt kind of silly. Easier to do with the mouth open, feels like it's hard to get the rhythm with the mouth closed. Going to ask my mentor more about this.*
Shītali/Shītkari	*2–3x*	*I've always liked shītali. It's easy for me to roll my tongue and the cooling breath feels good and relaxing. Since I'm familiar with this, it doesn't seem as challenging (or interesting) as the other practices.*

Developing the Tongue Chart

Week 1

Type of Practice	Frequency	Reflections on Practice
Jiva Mūdra		
Washing the Teeth with the Tongue		
Tongue Extensions		
Kechari Mūdra		
Clucking with Mouth Closed		
Shītali/Shītkari		

Week 2

Type of Practice	Frequency	Reflections on Practice
Jiva Mūdra		
Washing the Teeth with the Tongue		
Tongue Extensions		
Kechari Mūdra		
Clucking with Mouth Closed		
Shītali/Shītkari		

Week 3

Type of Practice	Frequency	Reflections on Practice
Jiva Mūdra		
Washing the Teeth with the Tongue		
Tongue Extensions		
Kechari Mūdra		
Clucking with Mouth Closed		
Shītali/Shītkari		

Week 4

Type of Practice	Frequency	Reflections on Practice
Jiva Mūdra		
Washing the Teeth with the Tongue		
Tongue Extensions		
Kechari Mūdra		
Clucking with Mouth Closed		
Shītali/Shītkari		

PRACTICE 5.3: DEVELOPING HEALTHY SPEECH

Learning to speak without over-breathing is a vital part of the breath-retraining process, especially for mouth-breathers. It's important to listen and hear whether your breath is audible as you speak. These simple practices can be helpful for teachers, salespersons, receptionists, or anyone who has a job that requires a lot of speaking. They are particularly helpful if you find yourself exhausted at the end of a full day of talking.

(A) Alphabet Practice

1. Take a gentle nose breath in. Open your mouth to say the letters a, b, c, d, e.
2. Close your mouth.
3. Take another gentle nose breath in. Say five more: f, g, h, i, j, k.
4. Close your mouth and continue.

You can gradually extend the number of letters spoken with each exhalation. However, always pause with your mouth closed and breathe in silently through your nose following your recitation. If you hear a gasp, no matter how small, you spoke too long.

Use the space below to reflect on your experience with the Alphabet Practice. Include the frequency of use and how effective it was in increasing your awareness of your speech patterns in relation to the breath and in transforming them. How many letters were spoken with ease? What did you notice?

____

____

____

____

____

____

____

____

(B) Reading Aloud

Similar to the Alphabet Practice, practice reading aloud to yourself. Keep your phrases short; even shorter than as marked by commas or periods in the book or magazine. The key is to observe your breath during and after your speech. If you find your breath agitated or feel the slightest bit breathless, cut your phrases to accommodate a quiet and smooth inhalation breath.

Allow yourself resting breaths between phrases whenever you experience breathlessness in this process.

Use the space below to reflect on your experience with the Reading Aloud Practice. Include the frequency of use and how effective it was in increasing your awareness of your speech patterns in relationship to the breath and in transforming them. What did you notice? What did this practice reveal about your usual patterns of speech?

(C) Mantra

Prāṇāyāma and mantra were traditionally taught together. The use of mantra to support the heart and mind will be discussed more fully in Chapters 8 and 9. In the context of reworking speech patterns to maintain functional breathing, you could use a favorite mantra in the same way as the Reading Aloud practice above. Let the breath cue you as to how long to chant. Remember to include a nasal breath or two, with a solid lip seal in between lines. This is different from working with mantra to extend the breath. The intention here is to make you more aware of and comfortable with breathing within your prāṇic limits, and not pushing into breathlessness.

Use the space below to reflect on your experience with the mantra. Include the frequency of use, choice of mantra, and how effective it was in increasing your awareness of your speech patterns in relation to the breath and in transforming them.

Note: Patience is required for re-patterning speech. Take time daily to slow your speech rate and become more self-aware of your saṃskāras. This will help you to be more comfortable with pausing when speaking conversationally or professionally. I recommend that you note your heart and breath rates, especially if talking for extended periods of time, such as when teaching. Accelerated heart and breath rate are indicators that the breath is pushed and you may be squeezing a few too many words in at a time. Practice allowing the breath to settle. Add breath pauses between your instructions: Close your mouth, and inhale softly through the nose before you continue with the next sentence or statement. The pauses will give your students time to process what you just said and allow you to calm your system down as you teach. Notice the effect on your prāṇa at the end of teaching with this kind of svādhyāya on your speech and breath. Notice the quality of attention in the room among your students. How have the pauses and the slower delivery of instructions from you affected their practice?

How has your prāṇa been affected?

PRACTICE 5.4: MOUTH TAPING AT NIGHT (PHOTOS 14 AND 15)

Mouth taping can be very helpful to curb mouth breathing at night, reduce snoring, and maintain CO_2 levels during sleep. That said, it is not always the most comfortable idea for people and may take some getting used to. The kind of tape matters. Use a hypoallergenic paper tape, like 3M Micropore Tape, or my favorite, Nexcare Gentle Paper Tape. If you don't feel any concern or fear around mouth taping, then proceed. Try different ways of taping to find what is most comfortable for you. For example, you may try any of the following:

- a horizontal strip across the lips
- an X across the lips
- small vertical strips across the lips
- a single vertical strip across the lips.

Apply a light lip balm to your lips prior to putting the tape in place. Pull your lips in, so the tape is in contact with your skin rather than your lips. Fold over one end of the tape (or both) to make a tab that is easy to pull when you remove the tape in the morning. In the first week or two, when you are adjusting to the mouth tape, you may awaken to find the tape stuck to your finger, your pillow, or your bed-stand. It is fairly common for people to discover in the morning that they have removed the tape unconsciously while sleeping. This is part of the acclimation process as your body and brain are getting used to nose breathing. Stay with it. I'd recommend cutting a couple of extra slices of tape and prepping them on your bed-stand, so if you do wake up mid-sleep and are tapeless, you can reapply another strip without fuss.

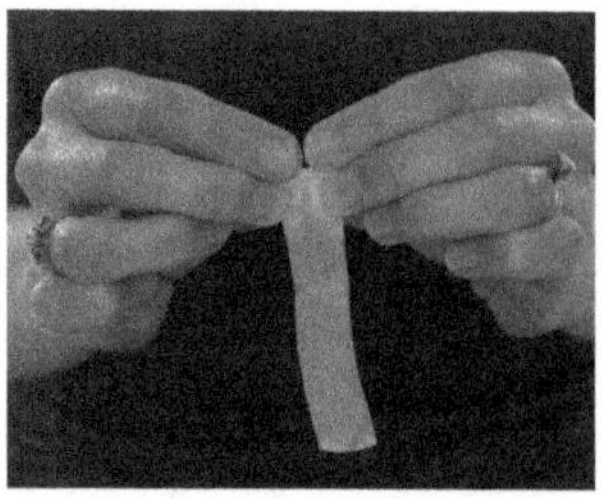

Photo 14

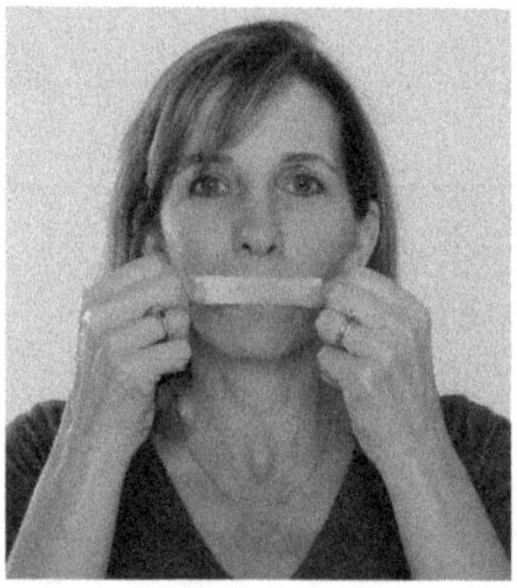

Photo 15

Ways to Build Your Tape Tolerance

You may need a little more support in building your tolerance and overcoming the feeling of anxiety associated with taping. Here are a few suggestions my students have found useful:

- Choose a few 20–30-minute daytime activities and wear the tape to get used to the feel of it. Washing dishes, folding laundry, watching TV, or even sitting at the computer are just a few suggestions. Any activity that does not require you to eat or talk is fair game.

- If 20 minutes feels like too long to start with, begin with 10 minutes.
- Be sure to make the fold-over tab that allows for easy removal of the tape, to avoid any delay when you feel the need to take it off. Gradually build your comfort level with the tape.
- You can also tape during a daytime nap or yoga practices: prāṇāyāma, meditation practice, or even āsana. If you have a habit of exhaling through your mouth during your exercise or yoga practice, this will help you to break that habit, while also getting used to the tape and higher levels of CO_2.

Use the space below to reflect on your experience with mouth taping. Include the frequency of use and how you experienced the mouth taping over the course of time. If you had difficulty in keeping the tape on or had to work through anxiety or ambivalence with taping, reflect on what helped you to move through your resistance. If you were unable to work through the challenge, note what you learned about yourself in the process of attempting this practice.

Taping precautions: Do not tape after heavy alcohol consumption. If you plan to use taping with kids, please see Chapter 5 in *Restoring Prāṇa* and follow the instructions carefully.

6

THE DIAPHRAGM, THE BREATH, AND THE CORE

The discussion of biomechanics which began in Chapter 5 continues with a close examination of proper activation of the diaphragm to support functional breathing. Differentiating between thoracic or chest breathing and abdominal-diaphragmatic breathing is the focus of this chapter. The undulation exercises described below are intended to help you to relax your neck, shoulders, and upper chest in order to temper your chest-breathing habit. Core Breathing—a variation on the Subtle Breath—teaches active recruitment of the abdominal muscles to support greater diaphragmatic action and core stabilization. Diaphragmatic Hugs and Push-Ups are intended to increase your interoceptive awareness of the movement of your diaphragm as well as develop resiliency of the muscle. The practices associated within this section of the book are very much on-the-mat, embodied practices. As you explore the relationship between breath and movement in your body, here are a few of the most salient facts regarding the biomechanics of breathing to keep in mind.

The Diaphragm: Center Stage

The diaphragm is most often touted for its role as the primary muscle of respiration. However, the diaphragm also acts as a visceral muscle representing a central meeting point for the cardiovascular, digestive, immune, urinary, musculoskeletal, and autonomic nervous systems. Consistent and correct movement of the diaphragm helps to maintain our overall physiological health. Additionally, the diaphragm works synergistically with the deep abdominal muscles to provide core stability, acting as a primary stabilizer for the lower back. When breathing is abdominal-diaphragmatically driven, it is considered functional. This means that at rest and during light activity, the muscles of the chest (specifically, the pecs, upper trapezius, and scalenes) remain passive. These accessory breathing muscles are in essence our "reserves," and are naturally recruited in the case of physical exertion like running up a hill or weight training, or in times of emotional stress to support the vocalization of a call for help.

Why How We Breathe Matters

The diaphragm is a multi-dimensional, parachute-shaped muscle, uniquely positioned in the center of our torso. It simultaneously divides and connects the thoracic and abdominal cavities. The heart perches directly on top of the central tendon or dome, and is enshrouded in the fascial sheath of the pericardium, which provides a seamless link from the diaphragm to the heart. Ensconced within the diaphragm, in the cave of the ribs, sit the visceral organs: the stomach, liver, spleen (see Figure 6.1), and hidden behind those, the pancreas, gallbladder, and kidneys.

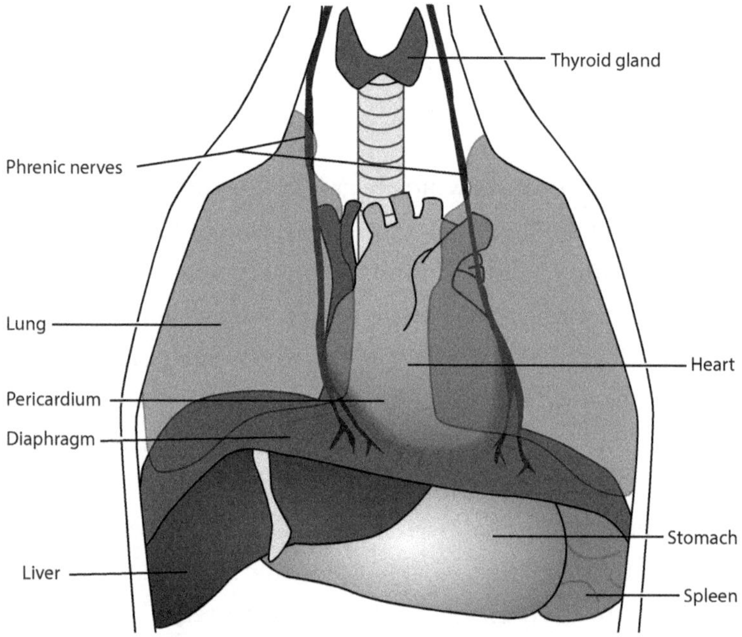

Figure 6.1 The Diaphragm and Organs

The aorta, vena cava, and esophagus bisect the diaphragm, supplying blood flow and nourishment to the whole body. Optimal function of each of these integral structures depends on the rhythmic pump of the diaphragm with every intake and outtake of breath. The costal regions around the edges of the diaphragm attach to the rib cage, and the crura (the long spindly fingers) embrace the lumbar vertebra, providing structural stability. The psoas and quadratus lumborum attach directly to the back base of the diaphragm and are part of a contiguous fascial chain which connects breathing to fundamental movements like walking, running, and lifting (see Figure 6.2).

Inhalation recruits the diaphragm actively. With each inhalation the costal fibers contract, expanding the rib cage outward, and subsequently flatten the dome. This creates a vacuum in the thoracic region, allowing air to enter the lungs. The movement of exhalation is referred to as a "passive recoil." The costal fibers relax, drawing the ribs inward, and the diaphragm rests back into its domed position in the apex of the sternum. If you have ever watched a jelly fish move, it mimics the shape and action of the diaphragm: The outward flare at the bottom of the mushroom head mirrors inhalation, while the inward squeeze mimics exhalation. Consider, for a moment, the health implications of this pervasive pumping force that the diaphragm provides 15,000–20,000 times per day as we unconsciously breathe our way through life.

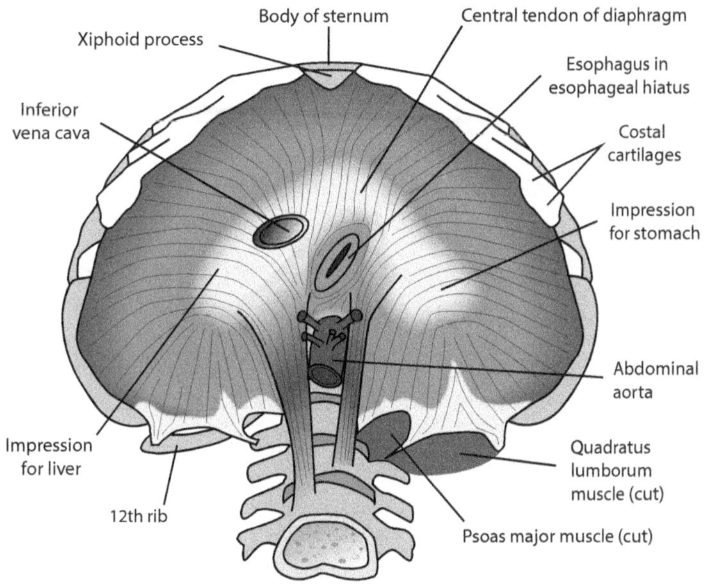

Figure 6.2 The Diaphragm

Abdominal-Diaphragmatic Breathing

In order for the diaphragm to fully participate in this critical action, the abdominal muscles which also attach to the rib cage are required to synchronize with it. When these abdominal muscles, specifically the transverse abdominus and the obliques, contract, they narrow the lower rib cage inward, thus augmenting the diaphragm's exhalation movement. When they stretch, they widen the ribs circumferentially, supporting inhalation. Conscious recruitment of these muscles to work in tandem with the breath reinforces diaphragmatic movement and gives us agency over our breathing in ways that enhance health (see Figure 6.3).

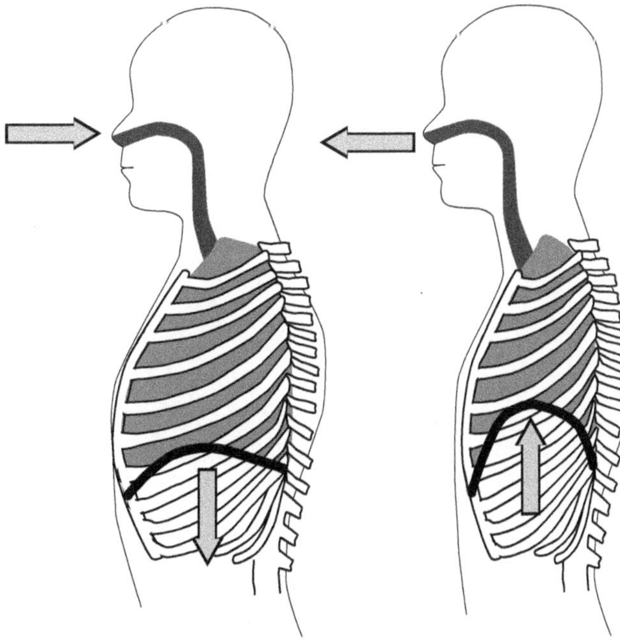

Figure 6.3 Basic Breathing Mechanics

Breathing pattern disorders, such as mouth, chest, paradoxical (reverse), and belly breathing, tend to lead to a dysregulation between the diaphragm and the abdominal core. Each of these interferes with proper abdominal-diaphragmatic recruitment. Chest breathing is the most pervasive and is noted by an up–down rather than out–in movement with the breath. The accessory muscles of the chest tend to over-engage, and chronic neck, shoulder, and jaw pain are often the result (Photo 16). When the muscles of the chest act as primary rather than secondary "breathers," the abdominal muscles become slack, and the diaphragm loses potency. Both chest and paradoxical breathing have been linked to an increase in sympathetic nervous system activation, triggering a circuitry of stress messaging from the body to the brain and back again. In paradoxical breathing, as with chest breathing, the muscles of the upper torso are held taut and lifted. However, the diaphragm moves inward and up, with inhalation fixing it in place (see Figure 6.4).

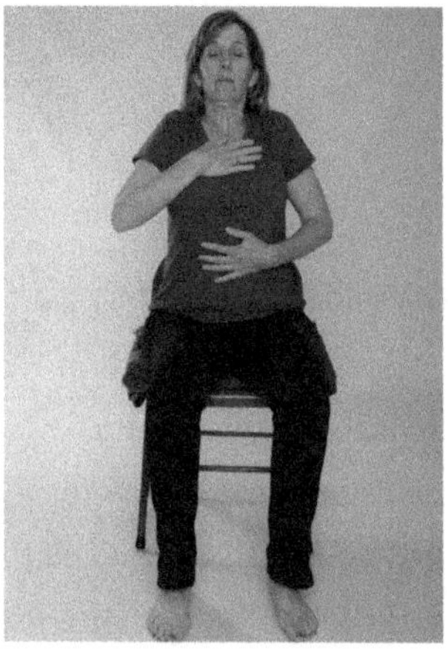

Photo 16 Chest Breathing

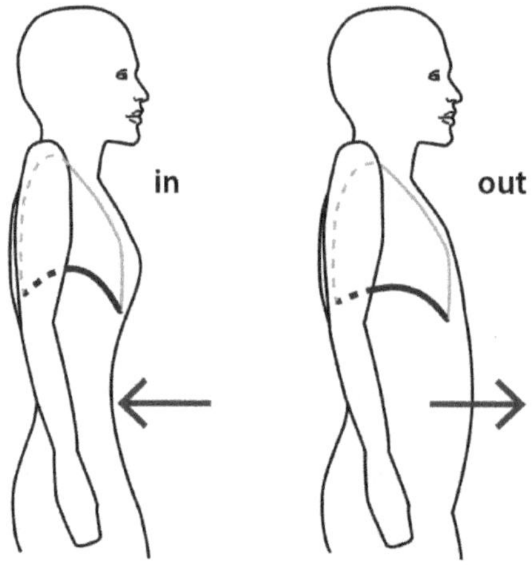

Figure 6.4 Paradoxical Breathing

Paradoxical breathing is often associated with trauma as it restricts the range of diaphragmatic movement, much like an animal playing dead to avoid a predator. Conversely, belly breathing actively stretches the abdominal muscles on inhale, but leaves them passive and flaccid on the exhale. In the short term, this is more parasympathetically driven and can have a soothing effect. It can be a useful means to reduce chest or paradoxical breathing. Over time, however, it inhibits proper recruitment of the abdominals. Consistent use of belly breathing prohibits the dynamic power of core stabilization that is provided when exhalation and active contraction of the abdominals are combined (see Figure 6.5).

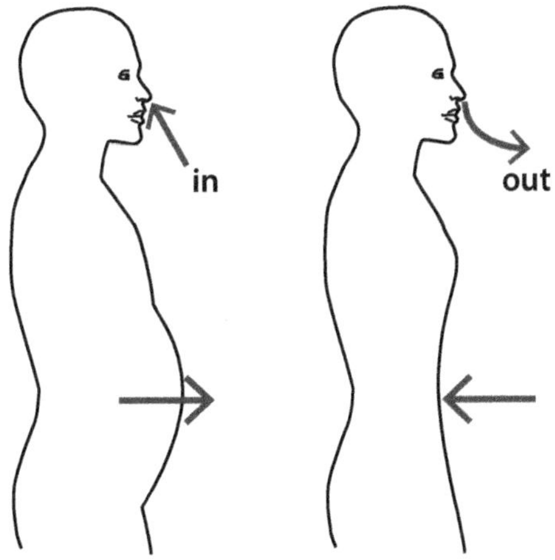

Figure 6.5 Belly Breathing

The Zone of Apposition

The *zone of apposition* (ZOA) is the vertical difference between the diaphragm in its domed, resting position at the end of the exhale and its horizontal position when fully contracted with inhale, and is used to assess the efficiency of diaphragmatic action. A greater differential between the two indicates a healthier ZOA and reflects freer, fuller movement of the diaphragm (see Figure 6.6).

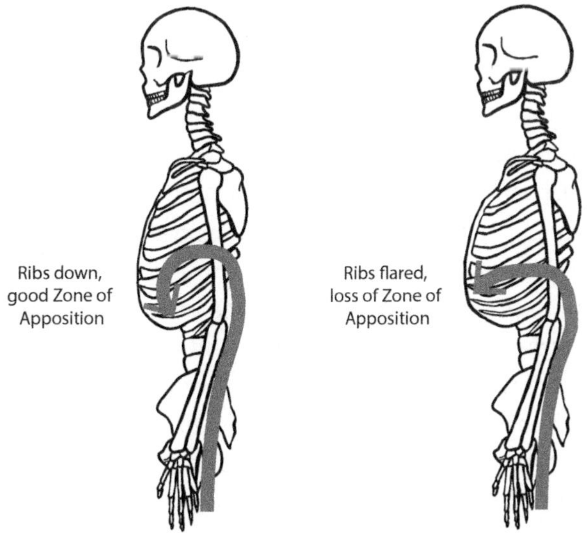

Figure 6.6 Zone of Apposition

A strong ZOA signifies that the diaphragm actively synchs with the abdominal muscles and is utilized as a core stabilizer. In conditions such as COPD and asthma, the ZOA is often significantly reduced, resulting in hyperinflation of the lungs.[1] Consistent over-recruitment of the chest muscles, relying on them as primary respirators, can result in improper positioning of the rib cage. This is reflected in the ribs protruding forward, as happens with spinal hyperextension, or in rib collapse, which occurs with slumping. Both the rib-jut and slump positions restrict the ZOA by impeding activation of the abdominals to augment full movement of the diaphragm. Chronic emotional distress or trauma can have a similar impact on the ZOA and is associated with dysfunctional breathing. Multiple studies have correlated good ZOA with core strength and functional breathing (that is, proper abdominal-diaphragmatic patterning and longer breath-hold times). These studies substantiate that when breathing and movement are matched in ways that maximize the ZOA, risk of injury is reduced and chronic pain, particularly in areas such as the sacroiliac joint, lower back, neck, jaw, head, and shoulders can be diminished.[2]

FINDING YOUR ZOA

To have a sense of the ZOA in your own body, try this experiment. Sit or stand in Tadāsana (Mountain Pose). Place the thumb and middle finger of one hand to touch both sides of the rib cage simultaneously (Photos 17 and 18). Intentionally hyperextend your lumbar spine so that the ribs push forward and the front of the rib cage is elevated relative to the back side. Hold this position while taking a diaphragmatic breath. Isolate the lower ribs and expand them as far apart as you are able. Feel the restriction in lateral movement. You may even feel the lower ribs pull in slightly, while the rib cage lifts. Notice expansion of the upper chest and gauge the level of tension in the muscles of the neck.

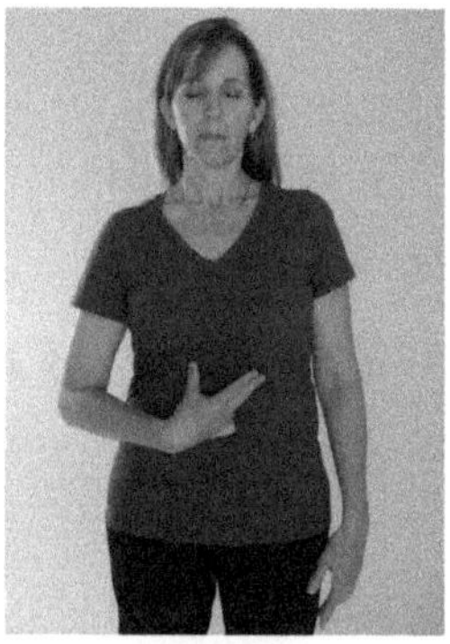

Photo 17

Maintain the hyperextension posture and exhale, engaging the abdominal muscles, hugging them in as much as you can without lowering the front ribs. Again, notice that your ability to narrow the rib cage with the exhale and move the diaphragm up into its resting dome is also restricted in the hyperextended position. Let go and take a few relaxed breaths. Now, tug the lower front ribs in slightly, so the front and back rib cage sits neutrally in a horizontal plane. (If you are a chronic "rib-jutter," this may initially feel awkward.) You may notice that the lumbar curve is also more relaxed in this position. With fingers touching into the lower ribs as described above, once again draw in a diaphragmatic breath. Focus on increasing the lateral expansion of the lower ribs. Compare your experience with the previous position. You should feel considerably less resistance, and a greater degree of global expansion around the base of the ribs. Activate the abdominals on the exhale and hug them in. Notice how much easier it is to narrow the lower rib cage. Depending on your interoceptive awareness, you may even feel the diaphragm moving upward inside the cavern of the ribs. Let go and take a few relaxed breaths. Now move into a typical postural slump. The lower rib cage will collapse inward, shortening the front waist, and rounding the spine in a C shape. Place your fingers once again on the lower ribs and do the experiment. Notice that the lower rib cage stays static and the abdominal muscles flaccid, unable to recruit with either inhale or exhale. The breath tends to move high up into the chest, becoming shallow and more rapid.

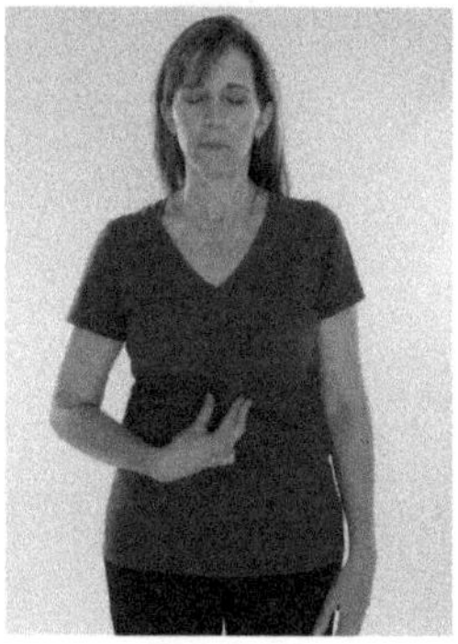

Photo 18

The Complete Yoga Breath

In the world of yoga, the construct of the complete or full yoga breath has muddied much of our understanding of what constitutes functional breathing. Unlike many other prāṇāyāma techniques, the complete yoga breath does not appear to be rooted in the Vedic teachings. This modern-day breathing exercise necessitates volitional engagement of the muscles of the thorax while practicing āsana and prāṇāyāma. In most yoga traditions, there is some call for chest inflation and an intentional focus on lifting the upper rib cage when inhaling. However, this method of muscle recruitment closely resembles chest and paradoxical breathing patterns. It tends to promote hyperextension, with the ribs jutting forward, creating tension in the neck, shoulders, and jaw. The trend to audibly exhale through the mouth during practice further compounds this dysfunctional pattern. Together these create fecund grounds for hyperventilation and postural instability. The exercises detailed in this chapter are intended to help you return to the ABCs of breathing biomechanics and provide you with a more informed means to activate the breath while practicing yoga (see Figure 6.7).

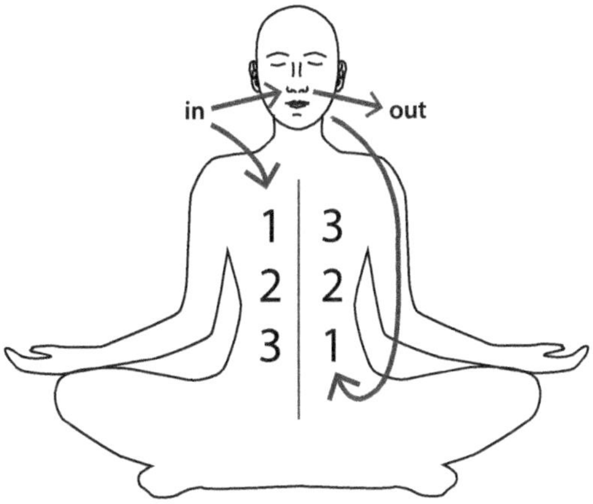

Figure 6.7 The Complete Yoga Breath

Preparing for Movement

The biomechanical building blocks that support functional breathing in this book are undulations and Core Breathing. Undulations are non-linear, exploratory movements designed to release tension. They help to gently mobilize and pacify the upper body while increasing awareness of subliminal holding patterns in the shoulders, neck, and jaw. Core Breathing builds on the Subtle Breathing described in Chapter 4. As per its name, Core Breathing consciously synchronizes the abdominal core muscles with the diaphragmatic movement of the breath. If you have difficulty finding, feeling, and activating the diaphragm itself, I have also included specific exercises to assist with this process. The practices in this chapter form the foundation for the recruitment of the *bandha* muscles as described fully in Chapter 7.

Note: The term *core* is most frequently associated with recruitment of the deep abdominal muscles. I have used the terms *mid-back core* and *neck core* as complements to the abdominal core, in order to link the pelvis, mid-torso, and neck in a stabilizing fashion. The abdominal core will be addressed here in Chapter 6. In Chapter 7, the mid-back and neck core will be detailed with practices, and the correlation between the core and the bandhas will be addressed. The combined and consistent recruitment of the "cores" assists both functional movement and functional breathing.

Undulation as a Pratikriya

Pratikriya, or opposite action, forms a conceptual foundation for āsana practice. Strong āsana traditionally was followed by a pratikriya or counter pose. For instance, Sarvāṅgāsana (shoulderstand) is used as a counter pose for Śīrṣāsana (headstand). Forward bends that flex the spine balance back extension postures. In a similar way, regular use of undulation provides a pratikriya for core work. Undulation is to be done slowly, with a quality of relaxation. It encourages gyration in non-linear, non-repetitive fractals of movement. Recruitment of muscles are performed at a micro-level, with mindful attention to every choice. Undulations prepare the neck and shoulder area for breathing practice. They bring awareness to chronically taut areas within the thoracic and cervical spine and instill a felt sense of release. These undulation exercises facilitate proprioception of patterns of tension while also providing relief. The soft swirls and rolls will help you to maintain a relaxed upper body, even while increasing the challenge in the abdominal core.

Undulation as a Practice

I often describe undulation as "claiming your real estate."[3] It has a way of enabling the practitioner to access places of "avidya"—unconsciousness—where they've not ventured before. In most āsana or movement classes, we follow externally directed instructions. Instead, undulation is self-directed, requiring us to use our own awareness to direct the movement to where it feels fresh. Like venturing down an unpaved trail, undulation beckons us to explore movement with curiosity, rather than sliding down a frequently traversed toboggan run of habit.

The rules of undulation are simple:

- Stay in a pain-free range.
- Keep the breath softly circulating without force or holding. Lips together; nose breathing.
- Move into "awkward." In other words, stay out of familiar "grooves" that feel easy and comfortable. Find new ways of moving: non-linear, unpatterned lines of connection that expose you to new possibilities for movement and simultaneously do not cause irritation to the area.
- Mix it up. Once you've explored a movement pattern two or three times, find another way into the area. Change the point of initiation, the direction of the movement. Add a swirl or curlicue that you hadn't tried before. Slow it down. Make it smaller. Refine your awareness as you "bushwhack" your way into previously unknown areas of your body.

Undulation increases circulation in the areas of focus. Over time it smooths out the jagged edges where the tissue may be adhered (glued together) or where there may be internal scarring due to injury or repetitive stress. In mobilizing connective tissue, it hydrates areas that have become desiccated from lack of movement. Sometimes an undulation practice results in a feeling of fatigue even though the movements seem so tiny and inconsequential. This is because movements that are unfamiliar require a great deal of mind/body concentration to sustain. Fatigue combined with a feeling of warmth, relaxation, and spaciousness are signs that your undulation movement is serving you. I highly recommend using undulation frequently before and in between the core exercises listed in this section and in the following chapter. Practice combining large and small movements. Choose consciously to move where you feel you need more awareness, a sense of spaciousness, relaxation, or desire to build new connections in your body. The following section gives instructions for specific areas of undulation for your exploration.

PRACTICE 6.1: UNDULATION SERIES

- Scapular Swirls
- Passing Notes
- Paint the Floor
- Doodle with Your Nose
- Forward Bend with Undulation
- Rapunzel

(A) Scapular Swirls (Photos 19 and 20)

This undulation brings awareness to the movement of the scapula (shoulder blade) itself, where many people lack proprioception. The key to this movement is to initiate the action from the inside (medial) aspect of the shoulder blade, maintaining passivity in the upper shoulder and neck. This practice goes far to unhook the upper traps, levator, and scalenes from acting as primary movers of the shoulder, arms, and breath. Many of us live as if our scapulae are nailed to the spine. Lack of mobility and poor positioning of the scapula is unfortunately a setup for anterior head carriage, shoulder impingement, injury, and dysfunctional breathing patterns.

Set your upper arm bones in external rotation as you lie in the supine position, with the wings of your shoulder blades tipped down and in (not pinched together). This will help initiate the movement from the bottom rather than the top of the scapular triangle. A slight bend of your elbow (as needed, use blankets or towels to prop your forearms and wrists so they rest comfortably) will enable you to link the back of your arms around your triceps to the muscles that move the lower part of your shoulder blade.

Scapular Swirls awaken the "mid-back core," specifically the serratus anterior, the lower part of the rhomboids, and the lower trapezius. Proper set and placement of the shoulder girdle requires functional movement in the scapula. To understand this more fully, consider how a skilled baseball or softball pitcher throws from the center of the spine, recruiting all the muscles around the shoulder blade both in the wind-up and the thrust. Shoulder movement that is confined to the ball joint (where the top of the arm attaches to the torso) lacks power and forces the tendons and ligaments to move the arm. The muscles of the rotator cuff and mid-back stabilizers are intended to be the powerhouses of the upper body. When practicing Scapular Swirls, keep your breath soft, abdominal-diaphragmatic, and in a continuous flow. Pause to consciously release any of the actions noted below which may indicate thoracic activation of your breath:

- subtle lift of your collarbones
- tightening in your neck and jaw
- jutting of your rib cage
- tension in your lower back.

Scapular Swirls are often easiest to learn in a supine position with your neck gently propped with a towel or blanket. The floor provides both support and feedback for the movement. Once awareness awakens, Scapular Swirls can easily be done in a Seated or Standing Mountain Pose, or even taken into standing āsanas such as Warrior 1 or Chair Pose.

1. Lie on the floor with your knees bent (you can support the knees with a bolster or chair, or have feet on the floor) (Photo 21).
2. Bring your awareness to the medial surface of your right scapula—where the wing of the scapula is closest to your spine. Practice moving just one scapula at a time.
3. Begin to lift, lower, and shift your shoulder blade towards and away from your spine (Photos 19 and 20).
4. Notice what moves your shoulder. Is it the muscles along the top of your shoulder around the curve of your neck? Is your arm moving?
5. Try to isolate the muscles along the inside and lower tip of your scapular wing, your shoulder blade. Imagine tipping only the wing of your blade in and out, up and down.
6. Notice if this feels challenging. The movement range will likely be much smaller if you keep it contained around the wing tip.
7. Feel your wing making variable contact with the floor as you move it.
8. Can you move in a different way (e.g. diagonally, in a swirl, figure 8, or in a random pattern)?
9. Notice where the movement feels familiar/comfortable. Notice where it feels awkward.
10. Move into "awkward." How else can you move in this area in a way that you haven't yet tried?
11. Pause and notice. Then repeat the practice with your left scapula.

You may find that one shoulder blade moves with more ease and awareness than the other. Use this side to "teach" the other side about potential options. Practice inviting the less mobile side to mirror the movement you felt on the side that moves with ease, until they are more congruent.

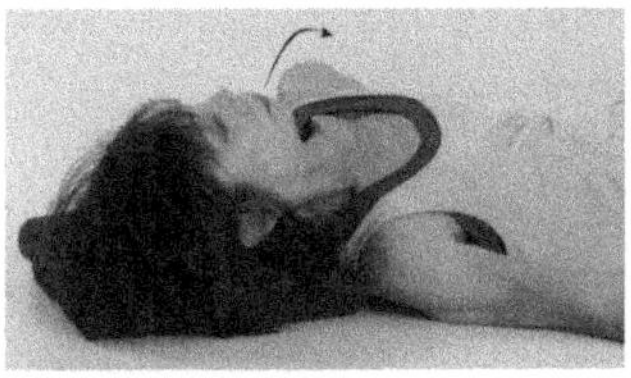

Photo 19

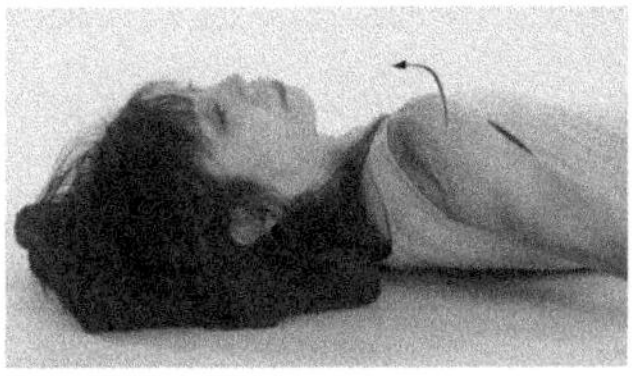

Photo 20

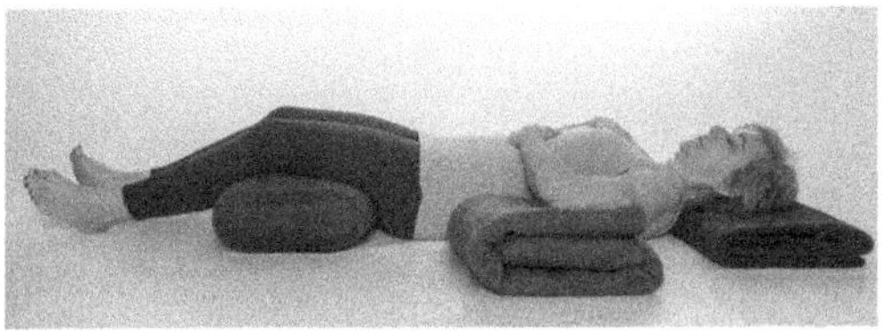

Photo 21

(B) Passing Notes (Photos 22 and 23)

Once you've become fully acquainted with the movement potential of your individual scapulae, alternate the action, right to left, as if passing notes from one to the other. Keep your neck relaxed, jaw soft, and your tongue parked to the roof of your mouth. Photos 22 and 23 offer a different view of the action of the shoulder blades while Swirling and Passing Notes.

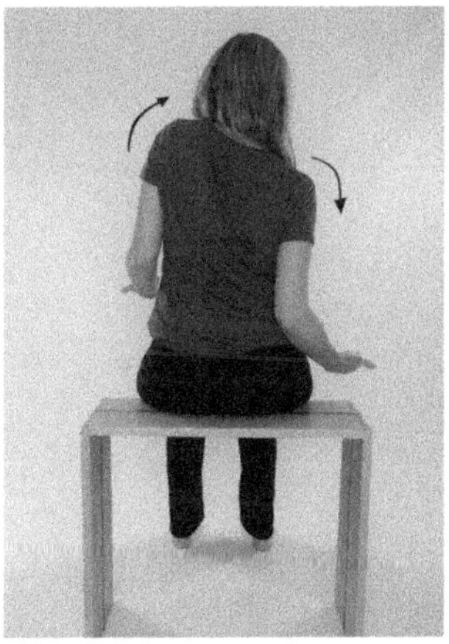

Photo 22

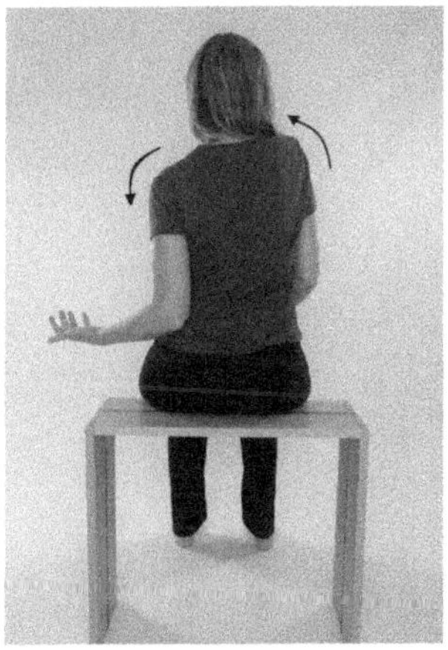

Photo 23

(C) Paint the Floor (Photo 24)

This undulation can be done from a supine position using the back of the head as a contact point, or it can be done in Child's Pose using the forehead as the contact point. The key to the movement is to vary it, so the contact point covers the widest "swath" of area possible.

Painting the Floor with the Back of Your Head

1. Lie supine with your knees bent.
2. Support your neck with a small cervical roll as needed.
3. Externally rotate your arms and set your shoulder blades down with the wings tucked in (not pinched).

4. Notice the contact point where your head meets the floor. Initiate movement from that point. Imagine that you are "painting the floor" with the back of your head. Roll it to the sides, up, down, and sideways (Photo 24).
5. Notice how it feels to change the contact point of where your head meets the floor.
6. Pacify your neck and shoulders with internal reminders to keep them relaxed.
7. Throughout this process keep your head resting on the floor.
8. Notice how it feels to tip down or lift your chin; to swirl your head to the right or left.
9. Explore non-linear movements, keeping the pattern random.
10. How much of the floor beneath you can your head "paint"?
11. Notice the effect of the muscles in your neck as you practice.

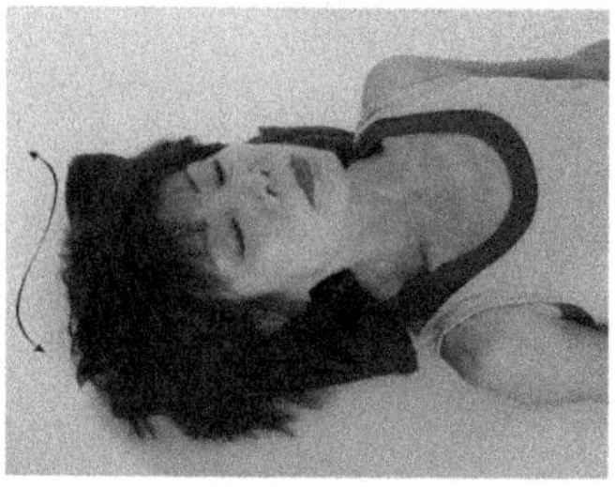

Photo 24

Painting the Floor from Child's Pose (Photo 25)

When doing this version of Paint the Floor, if your head doesn't rest comfortably to the floor, place a block or a blanket under your forehead, so that your head has firm contact with the support and your neck and shoulders can relax. This undulation can also be done from a chair (Photo 26).

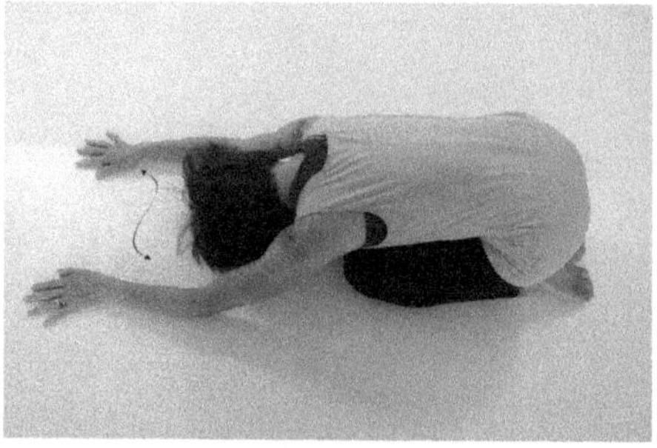

Photo 25

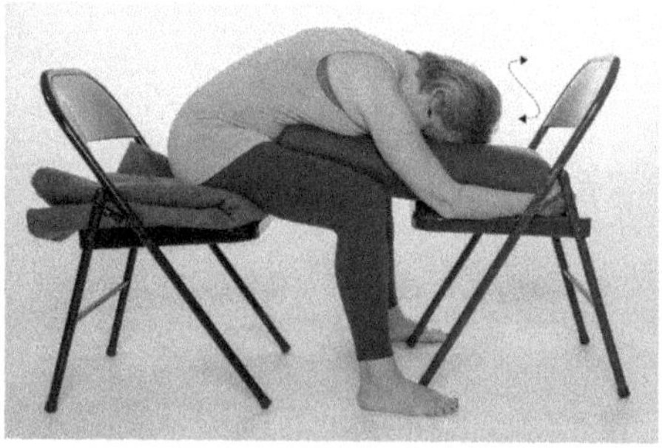

Photo 26

(D) Doodle with Your Nose (On the Ceiling or Wall)

This undulation can be done from a supine position or in a Seated Mountain Pose. It is similar to Paint the Floor; however, the initiation point of the movement is the nose. Imagine you have paint on the tip of your nose! Notice how different it feels to reference movement from your nose, rather than the back of your head. In a supine position, imagine you are doodling on the ceiling. In a seated position, imagine you are doodling on the wall across from you.

(E) From a Forward Bend Position (Photo 27)

These undulations can be done in Child's Pose, from a chair, or from a standing position as in Standing Forward Bend. Once you come into the forward fold, rest your hands either on a prop or on the floor. Isolate one area at a time and work with undulating that area, noting how it feels to move your neck and shoulder girdle in the inverted position. Scapular Swirls and Passing Notes are fun to explore in the forward fold to cultivate a different proprioceptive awareness than is possible in the upright or supine position (Photos 28 and 29).

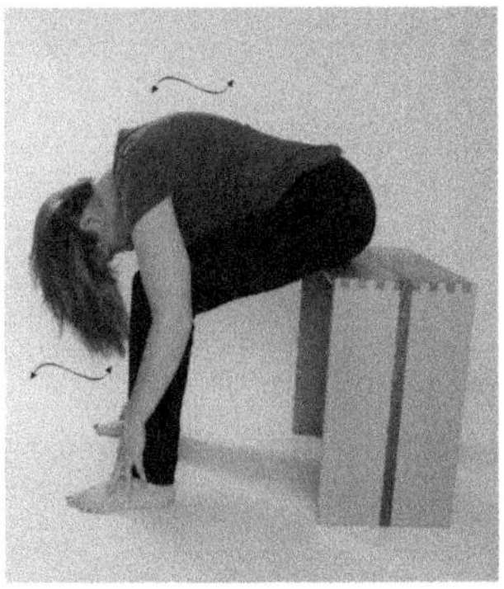

Photo 27

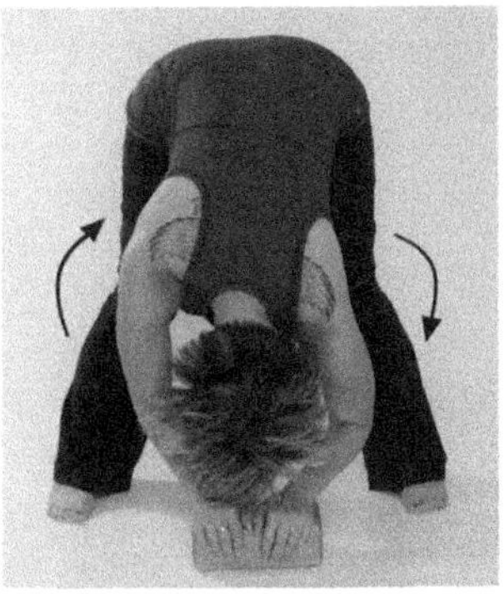

Photo 28

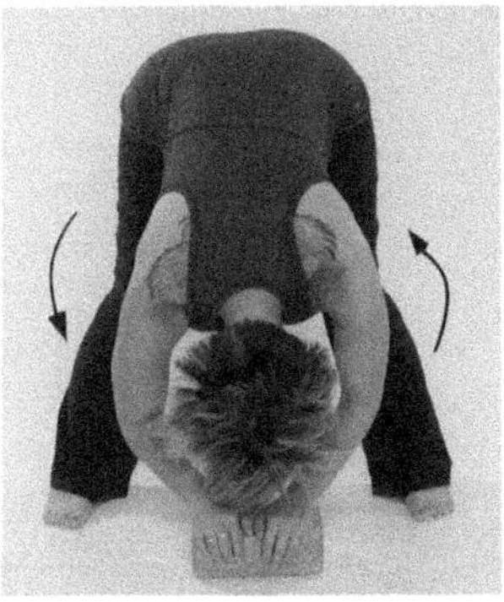

Photo 29

(F) Rapunzel (Best Done from Chair or Standing) (Photo 30)

1. Hang the crown of your head freely towards the floor, allowing your head to dangle from your neck.
2. Imagine you have a mop of hair that hangs loosely towards the floor.
3. Make slow swirls with the crown center, releasing and relaxing tension in your neck.

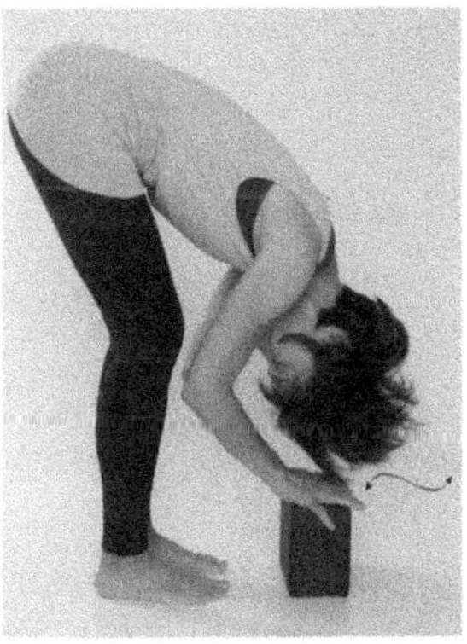

Photo 30

Intersperse any of these undulations throughout your yoga practice. They are an excellent prep for the stabilization and strength movements discussed in this and later chapters. They are also useful when you are aware of the tension building in the muscles of your upper chest and neck, or if you find yourself out of synch with your breath rhythm and striving with the inhalation. Let the undulations relax you and help you reset your body and mind, so the breath-retraining process feels inviting and easeful.

Journaling on Undulation Practices

Use the space below to describe your experience with undulations. Specifically address how they have affected your neck and shoulders and increased your awareness of areas of chronic tension, and how they have affected your breath patterns. Was the undulating movement smooth, or jerky? Did it change as you continued to practice? Were your right and left sides significantly different? If so, how would you describe the difference? Did you discover anything surprising in the process?

PRACTICE 6.2: CORE BREATHING SERIES

(A) Supine with Hi–Low Position (Photos 31 and 32)

1. Start supine with your knees bent, feet on the floor, a small roll under your neck for comfort.
2. Insert a block between your mid-thighs (not between or pressing on your knees).
3. Squeeze the block lightly to help recruit the abdominal core muscles.
4. Place one hand on your chest, one hand on your lower rib cage/upper belly (hi–low position) (Photo 31).
5. If your arms are uncomfortable or raised off the floor, use blankets or towels to prop your arms so your shoulders can relax fully.
6. Begin with Subtle Breathing.
7. Breathe softly through your nose, pacifying the muscles of your chest so there is no inflation of the upper rib cage.

8. Draw attention to your solar plexus; emphasize the outward flare of the lower ribs with the inhale and the gentle inward contraction with the exhale.
9. Take the time to consistently neutralize recruitment of your neck and shoulder girdle while inhaling.
10. Progressively make your breath lighter and silent, with less discernible movement (approximately 5 minutes).
11. Shift your upper hand to your lower belly, between your navel and pubis (Photo 32).
12. Maintain passivity of your upper torso.
13. On the exhale, begin to recruit your abdominal muscles by tightening the abdominals from your pubic bone, to your navel, to your lower rib cage. Imagine that you are zipping up a tight pair of jeans fresh from the dryer. Feel as if you are hugging your spine around the entire circumference of your waist. Hold the contraction of your abdominals for 2–4 seconds after the exhale.
14. Slowly, with control, "unzip" or relax your abdominals from the top down with the inhalation breath.
15. Repeat 5–10 times. Then relax the breath. Observe the effect. Repeat.

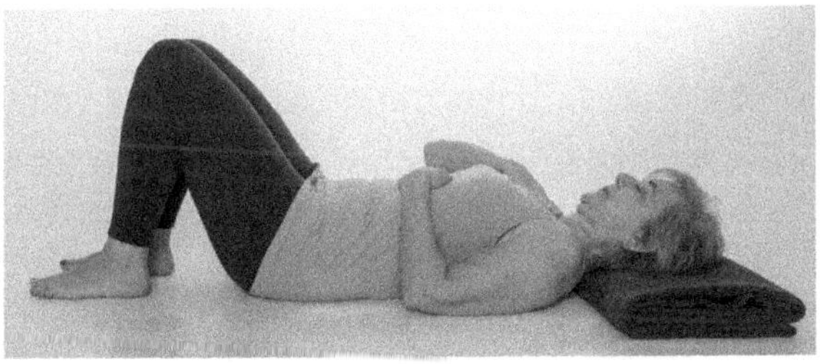

Photo 31

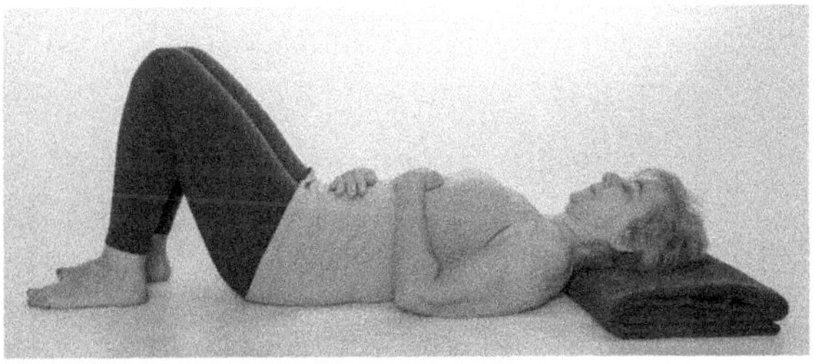

Photo 32

Note: When learning Core Breathing, it is important to attend to the slightest increase in tension or activation of your neck, upper traps, and pecs. If it is difficult for you to uncouple your upper body from this process, work more with the neck and shoulder undulations listed above. Then return to Core Breathing with this awareness. Sprinkle these undulations in between cycles of Core Breathing to reinforce your intention to maintain complete neutrality up top while engaging fully below.

Another common experience with Core Breathing is the unconscious tendency to increase breath volume to correlate with greater muscular recruitment. Can you instead maintain the Subtle Breath while recruiting your abdominals actively? It takes time to master this process but it is fundamental to carrying subtle Core Breathing into other āsana and physical exercise activities.

Tricks for Engagement

Sometimes it is difficult for people to feel the activation of the transverse abdominis (TVA). Here are a few ways I've found to help:

- As you lightly squeeze your adductors into the block, you will light up your DFL, the Deep Front Line. This is because the adductors are linked fascially to the TVA and diaphragm through the pelvic floor and iliopsoas muscles. Recruitment of your adductors can help bring your lower TVA on board.
- Try a pursed lips exhale. This is just for learning purposes—like using training wheels before two-wheeling it. Pursing your lips increases recruitment of your diaphragm and TVA. (Making the sound "shhh" works in a similar way.)
- Place both hands on the sides of your waist and use them as feedback for the expansion and contraction of your belly. First, actively stretch your entire abdomen as if you've just eaten a feast, inflating it into the palms—hold 1–2 seconds. Then actively contract the abdomen away from your hands as you exhale, zipping inward from the bottom to the top. Practice both movements synched with the breath several times.

A Word of Encouragement

For chronic chest or paradoxical breathers, learning Core Breathing may take several weeks (or even months) before it feels natural. Though challenging, it can provide a first step in instilling proper breathing biomechanics. Sometimes I observe clients getting the rhythm, then losing it. It flows and then it doesn't. This is part of the process. If frustration arises, relax your breath completely. I recommend using humor as a distraction, or doing a few repetitions of Apanāsana (Knees to Chest Pose) to release tension. Any of the neck and shoulder undulations offered earlier can also help reset your mind.

If you consistently find Core Breathing a challenge in the supine position, try it sitting up in a chair or work with the Developing the Diaphragm practices listed below. Some people learn through comparison and contrast. Exploring movement in a variety of positions, in different relationships to gravity, can often assist with building these connections.

(B) Core Breathing from Seated Mountain Pose (Photos 33–35)

Work with the hi–low hand position. First place your hands on your chest and diaphragm. Then move your upper hand to your lower abdominals. If tension arises in your neck and shoulders from holding your arms up, prop them as in Photo 35 to establish ease. You may also take regular undulation breaks.

1. Plant your feet on the floor.
2. Create a Seated Mountain Pose with your shoulder girdle set over your pelvis.
3. Elevate your pelvis using a firm blanket so you are perched on the center of your sit-bones and your knees are angled slightly lower than your hips.
4. Draw your chin in slightly, preserving the postural connection through your cervical spine. This helps counter anterior head carriage (forward head position).
5. If sitting in a chair, place a block between your mid-thighs (Photos 33 and 34).
6. Engage a light DFL awareness with your adductors.
7. Exhale and contract your abdominals, slowly zipping up or hugging in from your pubis to your navel to your lower ribs.
8. Inhale and gently release your abdominals from ribs to pubis.
9. Maintain complete neutrality in your upper torso throughout this process.
10. Feel for a gentle, lateral expansion through your lower rib cage.
11. Minimize any up/down movement of your chest and shoulders with inhalation.
12. Exhale and re-engage the abdominals, feeling a gentle lateral contraction through your lower rib cage as the exhalation culminates.

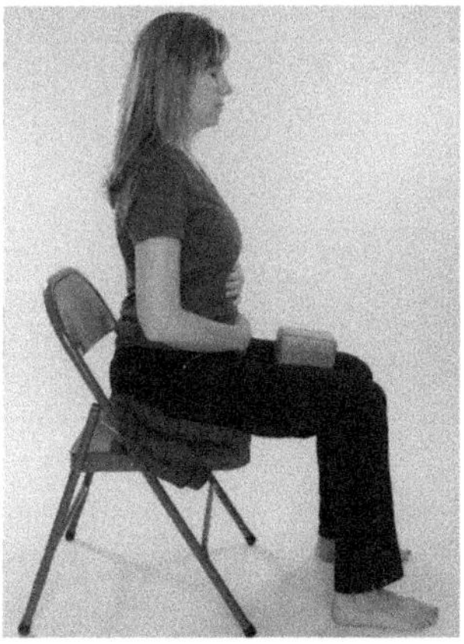

Photo 33

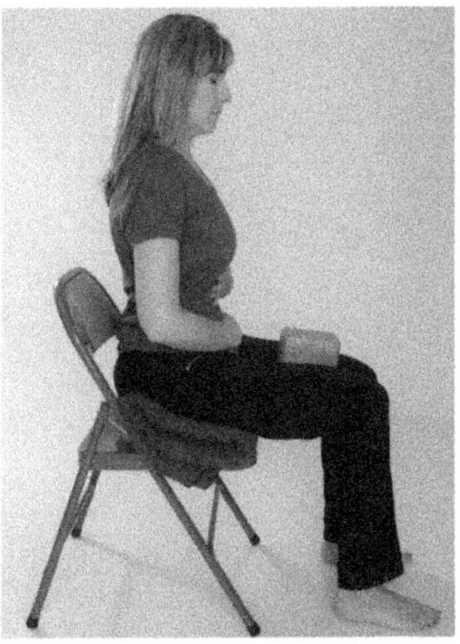

Photo 34

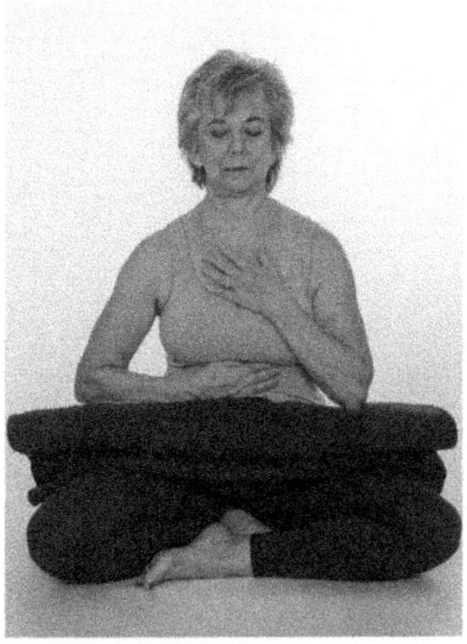

Photo 35

Note: Try a side-to-side hand position, with the backs of your hands or palms resting on your ribs. Sometime this position can quiet the upper traps and bring more lateral awareness to the movement of the lower ribs (Photo 36).

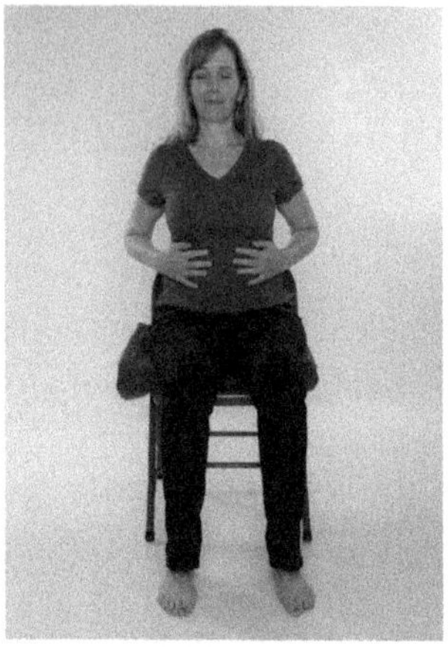

Photo 36

Journaling on Core versus Subtle Breathing

Over the next month, work with Core Breathing daily, adding it into your breathing practice and taking it into your āsana. Describe how it feels to work with the Core Breath and activation of the abdominal-diaphragmatic breathing in this way. Observe how Subtle Breathing and Core Breathing feel different and describe any challenges or observations that arise from this practice. Do you prefer one over the other? If so, explain why. If you find you are drawn to both, how do you decide which to practice?

Developing the Diaphragm

The yogis used techniques such as kapālabhāti and bastrika to activate the diaphragm and upper TVA and to move prāṇa dynamically. (More specifics on the traditional use of these techniques can be found in Chapter 10.) Use of these kriyas (cleansing practices) without care and proper guidance can lead to hyperventilation. At the same time, the pumping action can be quite useful as a conditioning and awareness exercise, provided breath volume is controlled and the movement is slowed. Synching the muscular contraction with the breath or isolating it separate from the breath can increase awareness of how to mobilize the diaphragm as well as strengthen it.

Note: In order to differentiate the traditional practice of prāṇāyāma and the kriyas named above with the practices detailed here, I have given these practices easy-to-remember English names.

These are best done in a Seated Mountain Pose. Align yourself as described in the seated version of Core Breathing described above.

PRACTICE 6.3: DEVELOPING THE DIAPHRAGM SERIES

(A) Diaphragmatic Hugs (Photos 37 and 38)

1. Place your palms on either side of your lower rib cage (Photo 37).
2. With a forced exhale, dynamically contract your upper abdominals (Photo 38).
3. Feel your rib cage hug inward with the contraction. Hold this contraction for 1–2 seconds.
4. Inhale slowly and lightly through your nose, relaxing your rib cage laterally in the process.
5. Repeat the process, progressively making the exhalation breath lighter and less audible, while maximizing the muscular pump of your diaphragm and upper abdominals.
6. When you feel fatigue, rest. Return to Subtle or Core Breathing and notice the effect.

As you work with Diaphragmatic Hugs, find a slow pulsing rhythm that you can consistently sustain. As you are able, pump in sets of 6–10 cycles, noting when the movement becomes asynchronous and your muscles begin to fatigue. Rest and relax for several breath cycles. Then, repeat 2–3 more sets, building stamina by increasing the number of cycles in each set to 12–15.

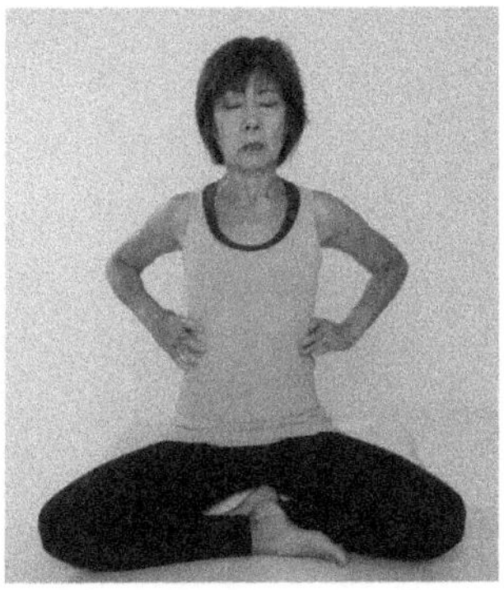

Photo 37

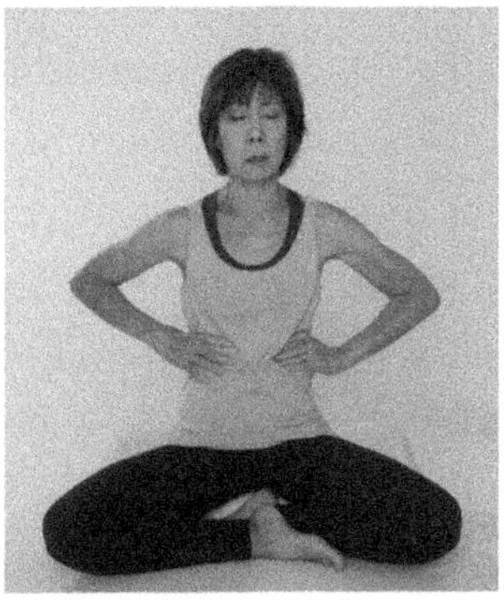

Photo 38

Note: The intention of this exercise is to synch the exhalation with contraction of your upper TVA and obliques, in order to increase your ZOA. If your chest inflates, or your shoulders lift, pause and do some of the seated neck and shoulder undulations suggested earlier. Return to Core Breathing or do a simple forward bend from a chair to relax your upper back and neck, and to reset your body and mind. The sound of the forced exhale through the nostrils can sometimes become a distraction. It is actually not necessary to create sound during this exercise. If you find yourself sniffing out strongly from your nose rather than initiating the action from your abdominals, this may be an indication that your accessory muscles up above are dominating the process. If this occurs, try the Silent Hugs detailed below.

(B) Silent Hugs

These are done on the hold after exhale or the suspension between the breaths. Silent hugs are similar to agni sara for those familiar with that technique. Silent Hugs are an excellent way to prevent hyperventilation and to isolate the movement of the diaphragm and upper TVA without having to synchronize it with the breath. Separating out these two actions can be especially useful for those who are new to this process or who have been habitual thoracic breathers with little abdominal-diaphragmatic conditioning. This exercise follows the same process as detailed above; however, it is performed without the breath accompanying the contraction and release.

1. Inhale and exhale gently and silently through your nose.
2. Suspend your breath (after the exhale) and engage your upper abdominals, contracting them inward.
3. Continue to hold your breath and pump your lower rib cage in and out laterally in a repetitive rhythm.
4. When you feel the urge to breathe, relax your belly and breathe gently in through your nose without force or gasping.
5. Take several relaxed breaths through your nose.
6. Repeat the process 3–5 times or until your muscles fatigue.

Note: Once your muscles have been conditioned through Silent Hugs, return to Diaphragmatic Hugs, activating them in time with your breath. Remember: The contraction inward always synchronizes with the exhalation breath, the expansion of your rib cage with the inhale. Pulsing your hands in time with the movement of the breath creates a powerful feedback mechanism that can be a helpful tool in entraining your abdominals. To do this, rest your palms face up on your thighs. Contract your palms into a soft fist as you exhale and relax them open as you inhale.

(C) Diaphragmatic Push-Ups (Photos 39 and 40)

This exercise uses the same pumping action as the Diaphragmatic Hugs, and can be done in time with the breath, or performed in the suspension between breaths as with Silent Hugs. Diaphragmatic Push-Ups, as the name implies, facilitate more active strengthening of the diaphragm. To do this exercise, lie prone and position your head comfortably, either resting your forehead on the back of the hands or on a folded blanket that allows your nose to be clear for breathing.

1. Place your awareness on your diaphragm.
2. As you inhale, expand your lower front ribs into the floor (Photo 39).
3. Feel your upper abdomen expand as you do this.
4. Hold the expansion for 2–4 seconds.
5. As you exhale, slowly hug in and draw your lower ribs in away from the floor and hold for 2–4 seconds (Photo 40).
6. Repeat 5–10 times or until you feel fatigue.
7. Both inhalation and exhalation actively engage your diaphragm and upper abdominals.
8. Rest and relax the breath in between sets.
9. Practice 2–3 sets per session, increasing the length of the pauses as you become able.

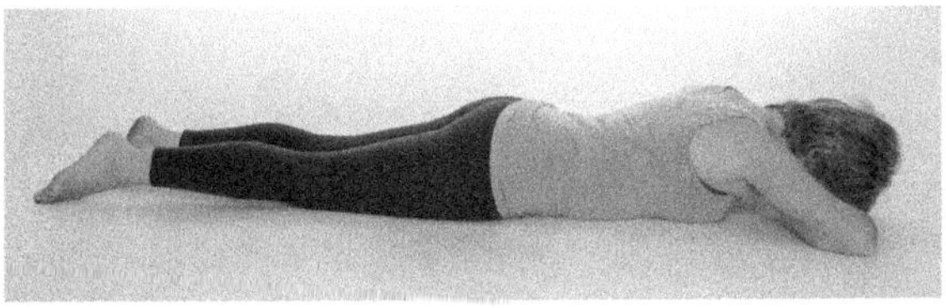

Photo 39

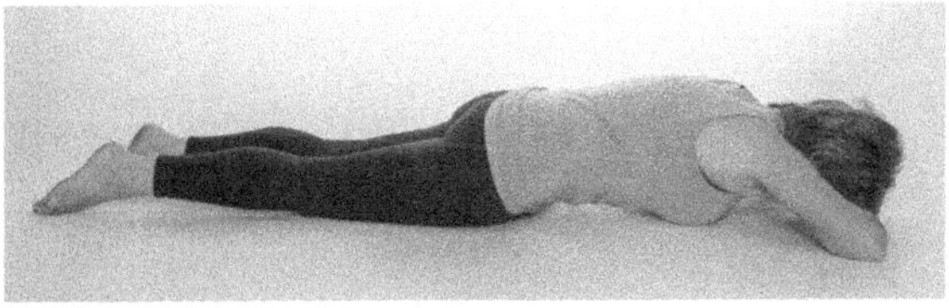

Photo 40

Diaphragmatic Push-Ups, as indicated above, can also be performed on the hold after exhale the or suspension. In this version:

1. Inhale, then exhale gently and silently through your nose.
2. Pause between breaths (after the exhale) and actively pump your diaphragm.
3. As you hold the breath, expand and contract your lower ribs and upper belly rhythmically. Feel your belly press and then draw in away from the floor.
4. When you feel the urge to breathe, relax your belly and ribs, and breathe in slowly through the nose.

5. Rest and breathe in a relaxed fashion until you feel ready to do another set.
6. Focus on the rhythmic repetition of the pumping movement, gradually adding more reps to each set.

Counter Pose after Diaphragmatic Push-Ups: Child's Pose with Paint the Floor Undulation (Photos 41 and 42)

1. Shift back into Child's Pose.
2. Let your head rest either to the floor or on a blanket or block so your neck is completely relaxed.
3. Imagine you are painting the floor or prop with your forehead.
4. Let your neck rock freely, and your forehead swirl in gentle, non-linear, non-repetitive patterns across the floor or support.
5. Allow your shoulders to completely drape, your arms remaining passive.
6. Move very slowly and consciously, alternating between larger, more open swirls and tiny micro-movements that release and massage the back of your neck and around your occiput.

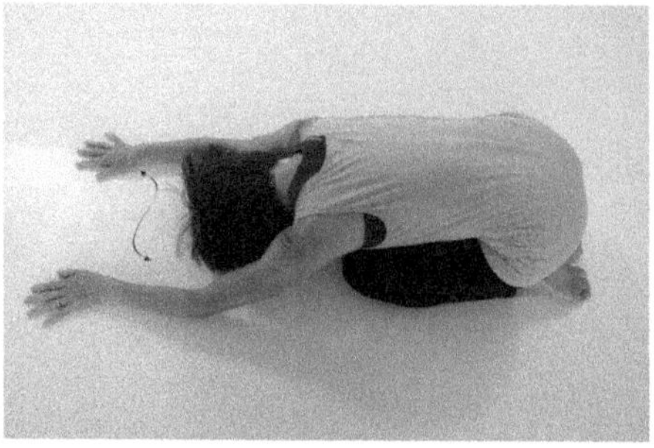

Photo 41

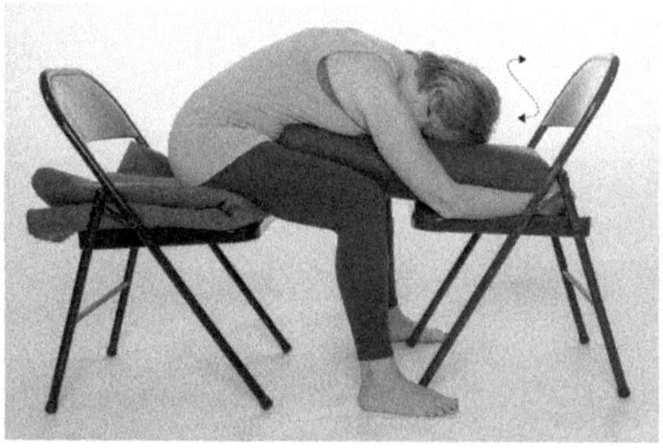

Photo 42

Note: If kneeling is contraindicated, this undulation can be done from a chair with your head resting on a bolster, second chair seat, or table top.

Journaling on Diaphragmatic Practices

Play with these diaphragmatic practices in your daily āsana practice. Notice how they impact your awareness of your diaphragm and your breath patterns on and off the mat. Describe any changes or challenges you experience as a result of these practices.

7

THE CORE, THE BANDHAS, AND THE BREATH

Traditionally, the ancient yogis used the bandhas—the root, stomach, and chin locks—to regulate prāṇa by manipulating heart rate, blood flow, and O_2 and CO_2 levels. Through their physiological mastery, they were able to sustain longer breath holds during prāṇamaya practice, which would induce the euphoria associated with the state of samādhi. For contemporary practitioners, the bandha muscles and their associated support structures in the mid-back provide stability, assist abdominal-diaphragmatic breathing, and help regulate the autonomic nervous system. Even without instituting a traditional bandha practice as in times past, the cultivation of these structures develops svādhyāya and containment of prāṇa in profound ways.

The Bandhas and Their Actions

Mūlabandha

Mūlabandha (MB), known as the root lock, engages the pelvic floor muscles and anal sphincter. Symbolically, MB seals the root center, thus preventing leaks, and supports the burning of ama (waste products) in the agni (digestive fire). The pelvic floor muscles form a multi-layered, multi-directional sling across the bottom of the pelvis. They are often referred to as the Kegel muscles, named after the doctor who developed strengthening exercises to decrease incontinence. MB activation strengthens the perineal floor and increases circulation to the pelvic area, providing an excellent means to address bladder control issues and prostate problems. Both pelvic floor strengthening and relaxation can be helpful to address sexual dysfunction, lower back stabilization, and, of course, good posture and functional breathing (see Figure 7.1).

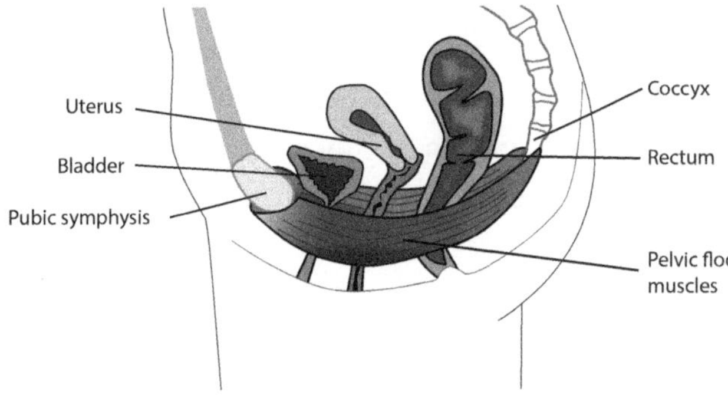

Figure 7.1 Pelvic Floor Muscles

Note: While traditionally the anal sphincter is a part of MB, when I work with the pelvic floor I encourage students to practice developing connection with the anterior (forward or front) part of the sling and to consciously relax the glutes and anal sphincter. This is, in part, because muscles that are used regularly have more nerve enervation. The anus and glutes tend to tighten easily for most of us and they will often impede our ability to feel the subtle layers of the pelvic floor. For more details on how to work with and engage the pelvic floor muscles, refer to the practices on developing the inner core at the end of this chapter.

Uḍḍiyāna Bandha

Metaphorically, uḍḍiyāna bandha (UB) carries the dross—the ama—up into the fire of the agni to be burned. Located in the samānavāyu (digestive center), UB is created by an intense contraction of the entire abdominal musculature (superficial to deep) which locks the diaphragm into the dome of the rib cage (see Figure 7.2). This pacifies phrenic stimulation and the call for breath, while assertively increasing the ZOA. Performing UB enables one to hold longer kumbhāka. UB is most often initiated on the hold after exhale, and held for several seconds to minutes, depending on the practitioner. It is then gradually released, before inhalation resumes. The intention with full employment of all three bandhas is to repeatedly engage and release UB for several breath cycles without releasing MB and jālandhara bandha (defined below)—a worthy challenge in interoceptive awareness for any practitioner!

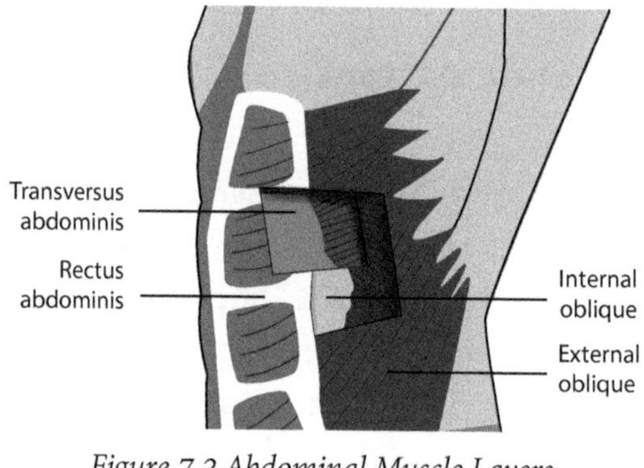

Figure 7.2 Abdominal Muscle Layers

UB provides great toning of the transverse abdominals and obliques, and develops congruency in timing of the engagement and release of these muscles with the breath. The intense muscular contraction and subsequent release around the organs of digestion, elimination, and reproduction are also excellent for healthy visceral function. While not to be practiced during menstruation, UB can be useful for some menstrual anomalies. Similarly, it can be useful for long-term digestive issues that involve congestion or constipation. For more details on how to work with and engage the UB muscles, turn to the section Developing the Inner Core—Preparing for Practice later in this chapter.

Jālandhara Bandha

Jālandhara bandha (JB), the chin lock, according to the Vedic teachings, symbolically locks the leak of divine nectar (amrit) from the "lake of the mind." On a less esoteric level, it helps maintain axial extension of the spine so energy can flow through all the chakras. JB engages the longus colli, along with the hyoid muscles, and the deepest layers of the scalenes, creating the "neck core" (see Figure 7.3). The neck core works synergistically with the primary thoracic stabilizers, or "mid-back core": the rhomboids, serratus anterior, and lower traps. The combined engagement of the mid-back muscles along with the neck core maintains a neutral positioning for the rib cage. This creates a solid vertical alignment of the shoulder girdle over the pelvis, stabilizing the upper torso and optimizing the ZOA.

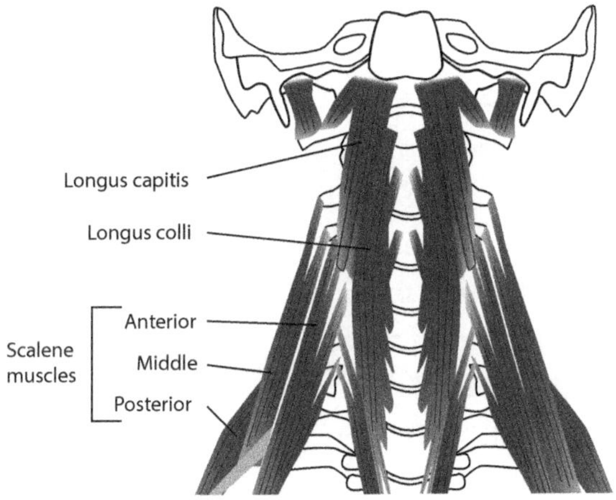

Figure 7.3 The Neck Core

Attending to proper placement of the tongue is a part of JB as well. With the chin locked in towards the throat, the tongue should press into a flattened position on the roof of the mouth. This action augments proper control of the breath. JB is initiated after inhale, then sustained throughout the prāṇāyāma practice. When JB is utilized for strong kumbhāka, the neck flexes deeply so that the chin fits into the sternal notch. This is essential for extended retention after the inhale to decrease pressure on the heart via control of chemoreceptors in the carotid arteries. Nowadays, this level of JB is not recommended for most contemporary yoga practitioners due to the societal epidemic of "text neck" that causes destabilization of the internal structures due to anterior head carriage. Traditionally, JB is held on all forward bends and axial extension postures, to keep the neck from either drooping forward or hyperextending. (See Figures 7.4–7.6.)

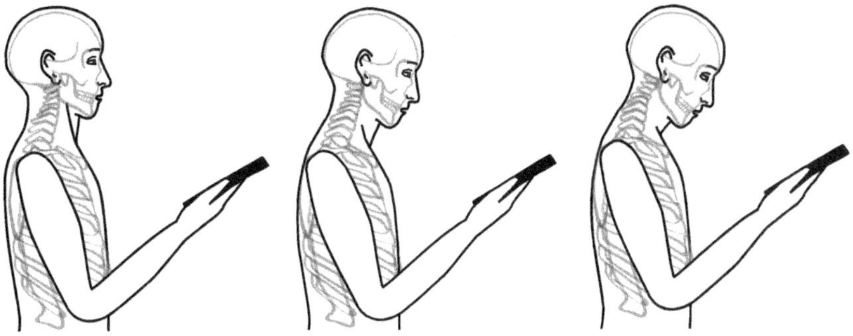

Figure 7.4 Text Neck

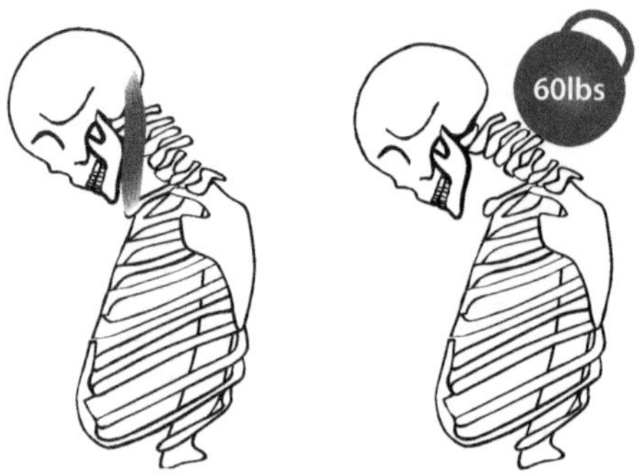

Figure 7.5 Traditional JB versus Modern Anterior Head Posture

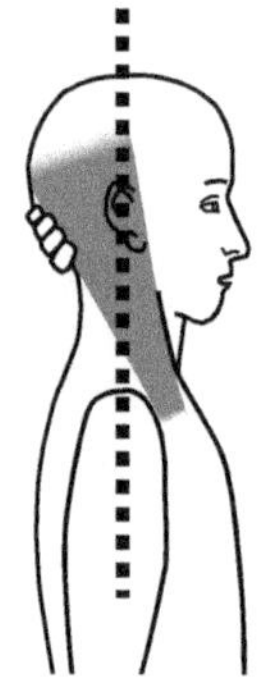

Figure 7.6 Neck Core Engagement without Forward Flexion

The Bandhas and the Core Today: The Deep Front Line

In his book *Anatomy Trains: Myofascial Meridians*, Thomas Myers refers to the inner core meridian as the Deep Front Line, or DFL.[1] This brilliant anatomy text outlines the myofascial matrix that holds our skeletal structure together. The Deep Front Line could be considered the inner batting that keeps us erect and in structural integrity. It forms a contiguous line of fascia from the inner (medial) arches of the feet, up through the adductors, pelvic floor, the iliopsoas muscles, respiratory diaphragm, pericardium, and through the longus colli of the neck (see Figure 7.7). In this way, a stable DFL preserves axial extension and establishes healthy postural alignment from the inside, supporting both functional movement and breathing. This helps stave off common postural anomalies like the classic "sag and sway" posture exhibited in many Western cultures (Photo 43).

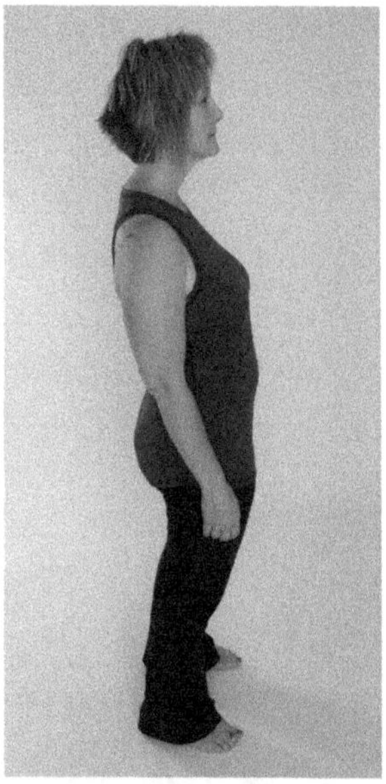

Photo 43 Sag and Sway

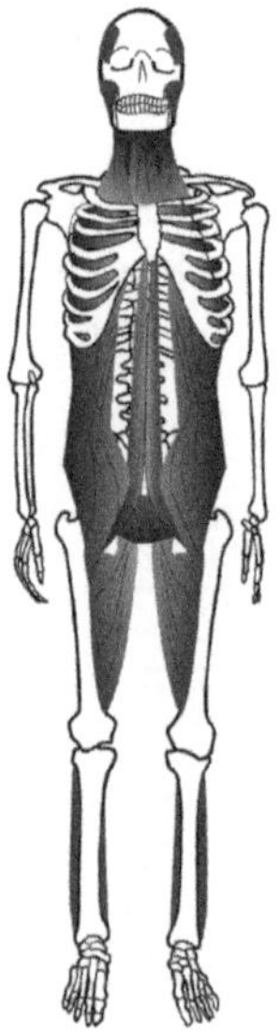

Figure 7.7 Deep Front Line

The transverse abdominis works synergistically with the DFL, meaning it assists with both diaphragmatic and pelvic floor activation. All three primary bandhas—mūlabandha, jālandhara bandha, and uḍḍiyāna bandha—engage muscles that are central to the DFL. Cultivating the relationship between these bandha muscles, the DFL, and the ways in which they interweave at the fascial level provides potency to both our prāṇāyāma and āsana practice (Photos 44 and 45). The development of the inner core/DFL muscles requires patience and a relaxed approach that incorporates a great deal of introspective awareness. The practices that follow build on those laid out in Chapter 6 for just this purpose.

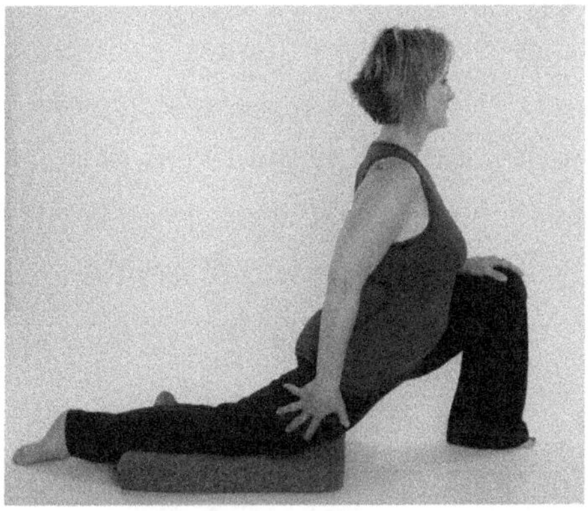
Photo 44 Lunge without DFL Engagement

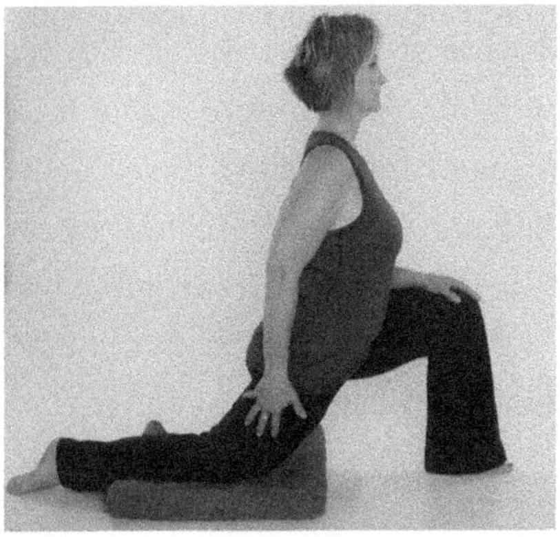
Photo 45 Lunge with DFL Engagement

Developing the Inner Core—Preparing for Practice

When learning to engage the bandha/core muscles, it is important to work slowly in small micro-movements, and to gradually hold the engagement for longer periods of time. This trains the inner core to function for endurance, rather than speed, and to provide stabilizing support for seated breathing practices, as well as facilitating the accomplishment of daily tasks with greater confidence.

Education of the inner core requires consistent reinforcement and integration, from the formative movements offered in this chapter into gradually larger and more complex āsana over several weeks or months. Building on Core Breathing, these practices tone and coordinate the bandha muscles and are extremely useful in addressing dysfunctional breathing patterns. The interplay of these biomechanical processes can shed light on how we can adapt our yoga practices to combine functional breathing with functional movement. This provides a stable foundation for our āsana and prāṇāyāma practices. Āsana in its versatility offers a multitude of ways to cultivate core stability, mobility, relaxation, and awareness, utilizing the breath and diaphragm as the hub of the movement matrix. When working with the practices detailed below, use the ZOA, or the neutral set of the rib cage, as your alignment compass. When lying supine, prop the head a little higher than usual to avoid jutting the ribs. You can also raise the feet with a folded blanket to soften the iliopsoas, allowing the lumbar spine to relax into a neutral curve. When recruiting the core muscles in the interest of breath retraining, we want to work slowly and progressively in a manner that supports endurance and maintains a quality of relaxation.

PRACTICE 7.1: DEVELOPING YOUR TRANSVERSE ABDOMINIS SERIES

The transverse abdominis (TVA) is a particularly long and broad muscle. It spans the entire area from the pubis to the rib cage, around the circumference of the body, wrapping from front to back to form an inner corset. Often people are stronger in one half of the TVA (either lower or upper) and rely solely on the stronger part for support. The practices described below are ways of identifying possible imbalance between the two halves and then using the divided action to "shore up" the weaker half.

When the ribs poke out, it indicates that the upper TVA is disengaged. A lack of lateral (i.e. side) gathering of the area between the anterior superior iliac spine (ASIS) and the navel indicates that the lower half is not recruiting. A number of issues, including back injury and pain, sacroiliac dysfunction, scoliosis, inflammatory conditions of the digestive and reproductive organs, and surgery in this area, can decrease one's ability to recruit one or other part of the TVA. Through utilization of the combinations and adaptations of the practices listed below, I have been able to facilitate the discoveries of numerous clients in successfully recruiting and strengthening their TVA. Always work with these practices slowly, synching the movements with the breath. Rest when fatigued. Build strength gradually over time.

Note: The question often arises as to whether the lumbar should flatten or sustain a natural curve when doing core strengthening. On this I follow the lead of my colleague, Staffan Elgelid, physical therapist, yoga therapist, Feldenkrais practitioner, and the author of *Smart Core* (one of the best core-strengthening video series on the market). Staffan states that we want our core muscles strong and flexibly adaptive to real life, not rigidly accessible in only one postural stance. With this in mind, you can start these practices in the position that you feel strongest; perhaps that means maintaining a neutral arch or a more flattened lumbar curve. You may in fact wish to prop your low back with a small hand-towel if you have experienced recent lumbar injury or low back pain. However, as you build more strength and awareness, I encourage you to explore various positions of the pelvis, rather than holding your back rigid in one position.

One significant note is that if your abdominals are pushing out and hardening as you exhale, you are not utilizing your TVA as the corset it was intended to be. Hollow your belly inward, as if making a little cup with your navel area. As you work progressively, moderate the load within a range of effort that allows you to maintain this hollow shape of your belly. This action always coordinates with the exhalation.

In the context of this book, the most important factor is learning to synch your abdominals and diaphragm with your breath, training them to work synergistically together. There is no need to add load or in any way strain or stress your lower back to achieve this. In fact, it is critical that you feel stable and able to maintain a calm, relaxed nasal breath as you work. Let the quality of the breath determine your level of challenge. If the breath feels pushed, or becomes audible, back off and adjust the level of effort to create more ease with your movement.

(A) Block Squeeze and 2-Part Exhale (Krama Exhale) (Photo 46)

The term *krama* refers to a stepped, segmented, or staged action. This may mean dividing a movement or a breath into fractional parts—for instance, halves, thirds, or quarters. Krama acts as a useful concept and technique for linking mind, breath, and body. It's a vehicle for cultivating svādhyāya, and for breaking habitual patterns. In the following practices, krama breath is combined with krama movement to bring more awareness to the upper and lower parts of the TVA, while simultaneously interrupting the "big breath saṃskāra." With all of these practices, keep each segment of breath small: between 1 and 3 seconds in length. Overall length of inhale will approximate 4–6 seconds; however, the intention of these practices is not to measure the length of the breath. Instead, practice "sipping" the breath and timing it with the engagement of your core muscles.

1. Begin with supine Core Breathing, with your knees bent, and your feet on the floor.
2. Insert a block between your mid-thighs (not between or pressing on your knees).
3. Engage a light DFL awareness with your adductors.
4. Place your hands in the hi–low position—one on your lower abs below the navel, one on your diaphragm.
5. Pacify the muscles of your chest as you inhale, and gently expand your lower rib cage to ensure more diaphragmatic action.
6. Divide the exhalation breath into two "parts," simultaneously dividing the contraction of your TVA into halves: lower and upper.
7. With the first half of the exhale, hug in or zip up your lower belly, engaging the muscles from your pubic bone to your navel.
8. Hold for 2 seconds.
9. With the second half of the exhale, hug in or zip up, engaging the muscles from your navel to your solar plexus.
10. Hold again for 2 seconds.
11. With the inhale, create a smooth, controlled release of your abdominal muscles from the top down.
12. Repeat 3–5 times or to fatigue, then rest the breath and belly for several minutes.
13. As you are able, repeat another 2–3 reps, practicing the 2-part krama exhale.

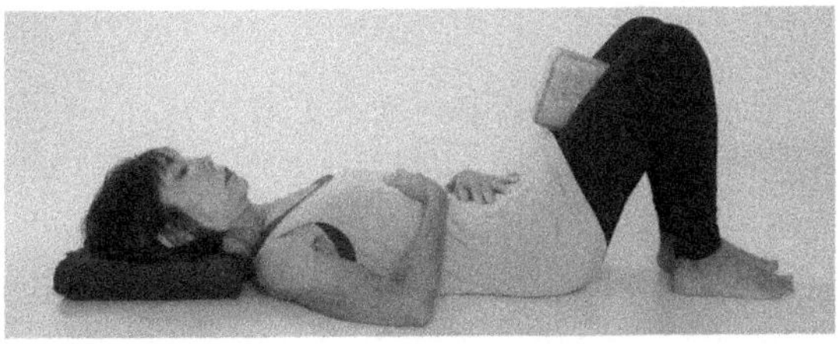

Photo 46

Block Squeeze and 2-Part Exhale and Inhale

As you become more proficient at this action, practice taking the krama in reverse (with the inhalation), releasing the inner zipper in two parts. This will combine the expansion of your lower rib cage with the release of your abdominals during the inhalation breath. Breath length will vary between 4 and 6 seconds, with the exhale slightly longer than the inhale. The breath should not feel pressured or pushed. Be conscious of the tendency to move into "rib-jut," or a slight hyperextension of your mid-to-lower-back, as you do this movement. Can you maintain awareness of your ZOA and keep it neutral as you do this practice?

1. With the first half of the inhale, release your abdominals from your diaphragm to your navel.
2. Hold for 2 seconds.
3. With the second half of the inhale, release your lower abdominals from your navel to your pubis.
4. Hold for 2 seconds.
5. Combine the 2-part inhale with the 2-part exhale. Work to fatigue. Then rest, relax, and observe the natural flow of the breath and your awareness.

This TVA practice can also be done from a Seated Tadāsana/Mountain Pose or even in Wall Sits (Utkatāsana/Chair Pose at the Wall; see below). With the block between your thighs, your adductors stay engaged, providing more DFL support from your feet and inner legs, all the way up the fascial line.

(B) Apanāsana/Knees to Chest with 2-Part Krama Exhale (Photos 47–51)

1. Place a folded blanket, towel, or small pillow under your neck and head for light cervical support.
2. Start with Core Breathing in the supine position (Photo 47).
3. Insert the block between your mid-thighs (not between or pressing on your knees).
4. Engage a light DFL awareness with your adductors.
5. Draw the chin in towards the throat, creating a gentle JB-like action.
6. Set your rib cage in a neutral position.
7. As you exhale, squeeze the block and engage your lower TVA; lift both feet off the floor.
8. With the feet lifted and your knees bent at a right angle, bring your thighs perpendicular and shins parallel to the floor. Keep your legs firm, ankles flexed (Photo 48).
9. Pacify the upper body. Stretch your arms out to the sides in a soft "T" (with a slight bend in your elbows). Turn your palms face up. Set your shoulder blades down, with the wings tipped inward.

10. With the first half of a 2-part krama breath, begin to draw your knees halfway in to your chest. Simultaneously, hug your abdominals in from your pubic bone to your navel (Photo 49).
11. Hold for 2 seconds.
12. With the second half of the exhale, continue to draw your knees into your lower ribs, hugging your abdominals in all the way (Photo 50).
13. Hold for 2 seconds.
14. As you inhale, slowly release your knees back to their starting/right-angle position and relax your TVA (Photo 48). (Do not bring your feet back to the floor.)
15. Repeat this āsana 4–6 times or until your abdominal muscles feel fatigued.
16. Consistently check in with your neck, shoulders, and jaw for tension. Undulate between reps as necessary.

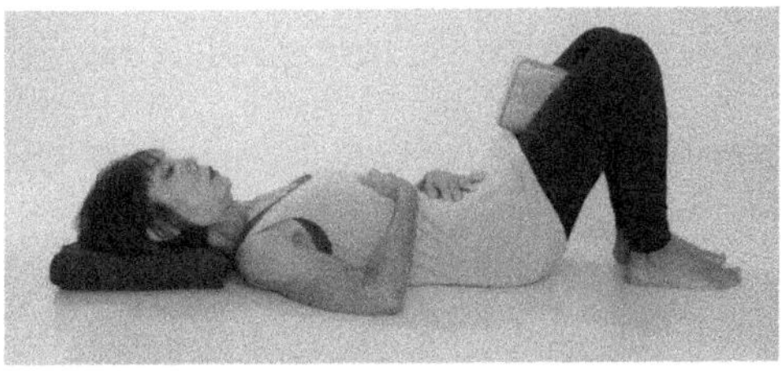

Photo 47

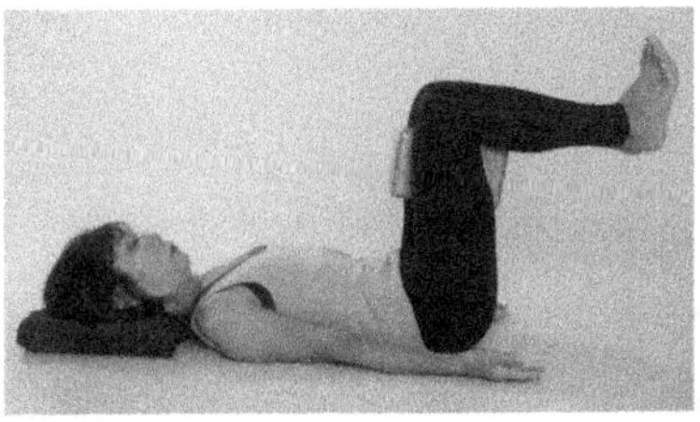

Photo 48

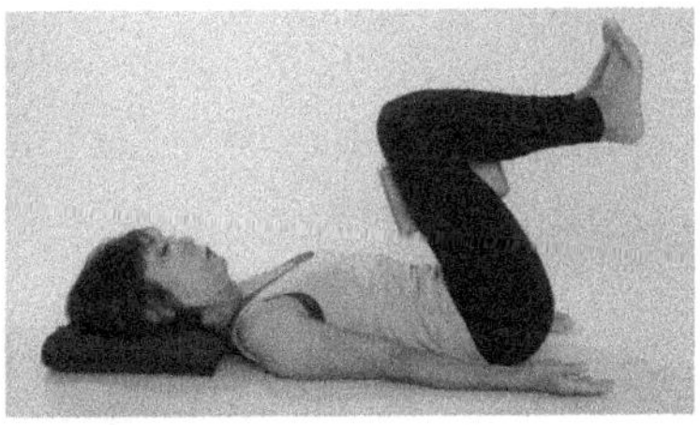

Photo 49

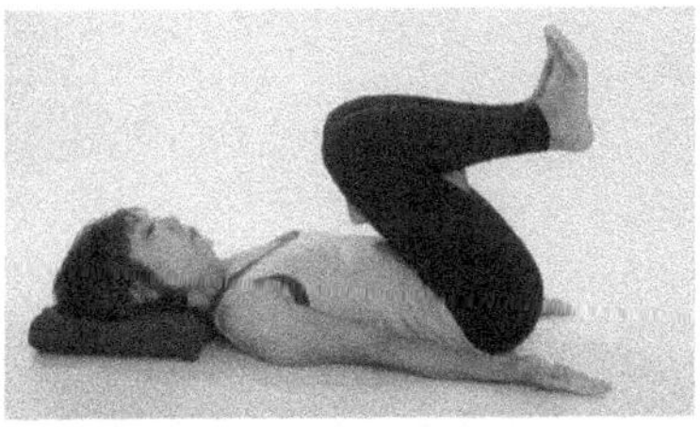

Photo 50

Precautionary Notes

- If your chin lifts at any point during the process, it means you have released the JB contraction. Pause and reset as necessary (Photo 51).
- Notice the set of your rib cage to maintain optimum ZOA.
- If your upper body is tensing, take a rest and undulate. Place your feet on the floor and try a few Scapular Swirls or Paint the Floor Undulations, as described in Chapter 6.

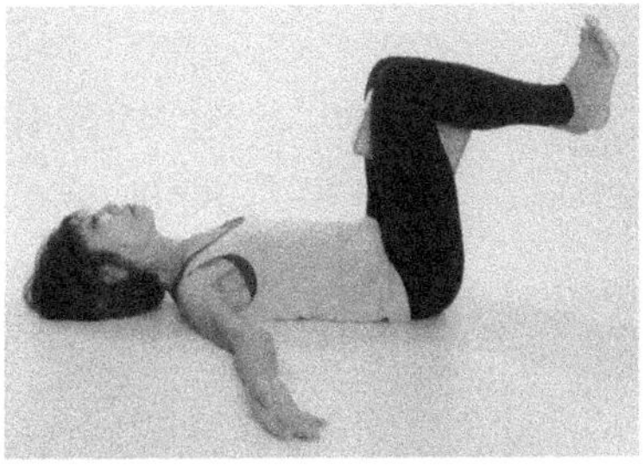

Photo 51

Variations: If your feet keep falling together in this position, try placing the block between your calves instead of your thighs. This engages your DFL at its roots, and often provides new svādhyāya of how the whole kinetic chain works. As you become more proficient with this movement, try adding a 2-part krama inhale movement. With this variation, you'll gradually release first the upper, then the lower TVA on inhalation as you move the knees progressively away from your chest. Maintain neutrality in the rib cage—ZOA awareness—as you do this movement.

(C) Bridge with Block 2–3-Part Krama Exhale (Photos 52–54)

1. Begin with supine Core Breathing (Photo 47).
2. Insert a block between your mid-thighs.
3. Engage a light DFL awareness with your adductors.
4. With the inhale, press your feet into the floor and lift your pelvis, stretching the front of your body (Photo 52).
5. With the first half of the 2-part krama exhale, draw your lower abs in and curl your spine halfway down.
6. Hold for 2 seconds (Photo 53).
7. With the second half of the 2-part krama exhale, curl your spine all the way down.
8. Hold for 2 seconds (Photo 54).
9. Repeat this āsana 3–5 times.
10. Return to Core Breathing and notice the effect of the practice.

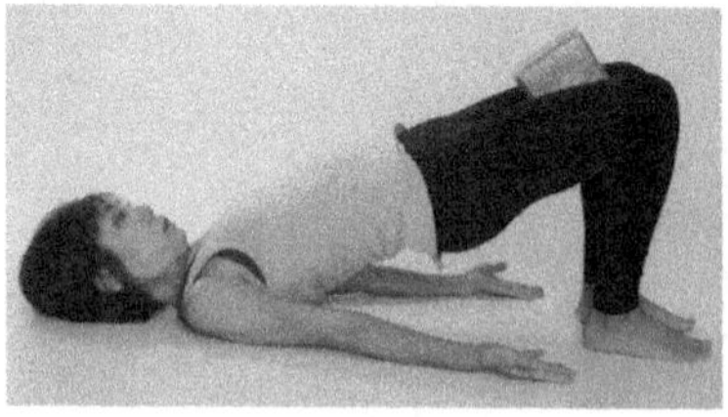

Photo 52

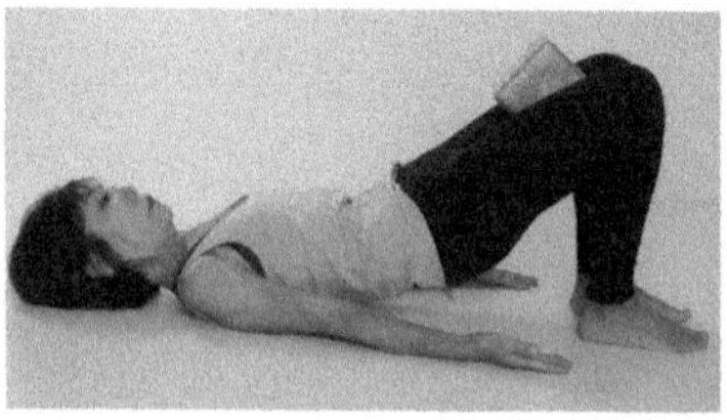

Photo 53

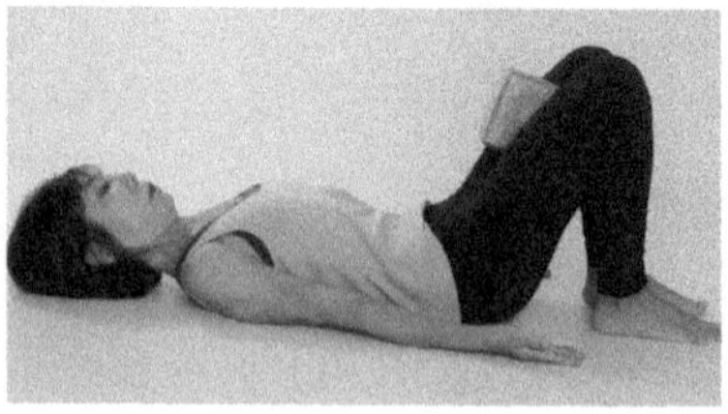

Photo 54

If you wish to work more intensely, try progressively increasing the holds to 3–4–5 seconds. Alternately, experiment with breaking the breath and movement into three parts, refining the activation of your TVA with a more controlled breath and while gradually flexing your spine. With all of these Bridge variations, maintain a steady squeeze into the block and firm pressure through the soles of your feet and up into your glutes.

(D) Chakravakāsana or Wheel Pose with 2-Part Exhale (Photos 55–57)

1. Position yourself in Child's Pose with your hands forward, shoulder width apart, your elbows soft and forearms resting on the floor (Photo 55).
2. With the inhalation breath, move forward into the spinal extension position of Cat/Cow (Photo 56).
3. Avoid hyperextension of your neck by drawing the chin into a light JB, gazing towards the floor, rather than looking up.
4. Avoid hyperextension of your lower back, by hugging in your TVA, thereby creating a safety net of support for your lumbar spine.
5. With the first half of the 2-part krama exhalation, lead with an even stronger abdominal lift inward through your lower TVA, and draw your hips halfway back towards Child's Pose (Photo 57).
6. Hold for 2 seconds.
7. Let your head relax and release. Allow your elbows to fold towards the floor so your thoracic kyphosis is not exaggerated. Relax your neck into a soft flexion.
8. With the second half of the 2-part krama exhalation, continue to hug in your upper TVA and bring your hips further back towards Child's Pose (Photo 55).
9. Allow your forehead and forearms to rest fully to the floor (or on a light support).
10. Rest for a breath as needed, then repeat the movement 3–5 more times.

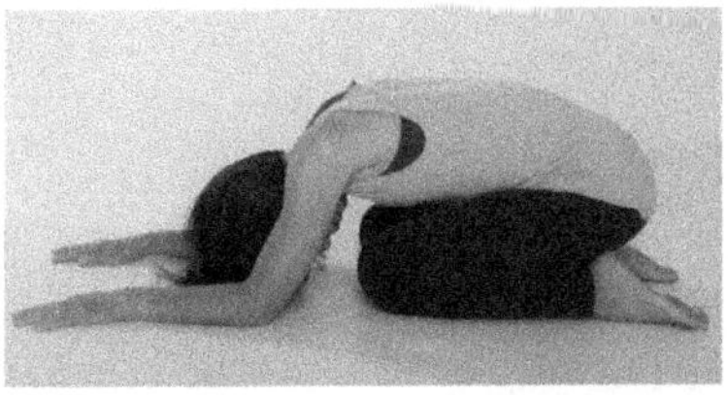

Photo 55

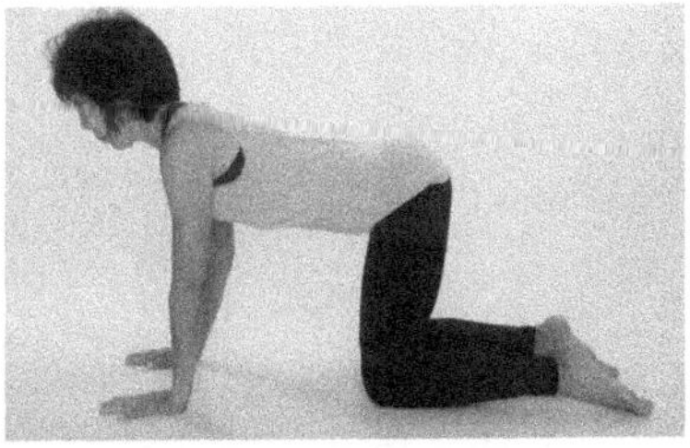

Photo 56

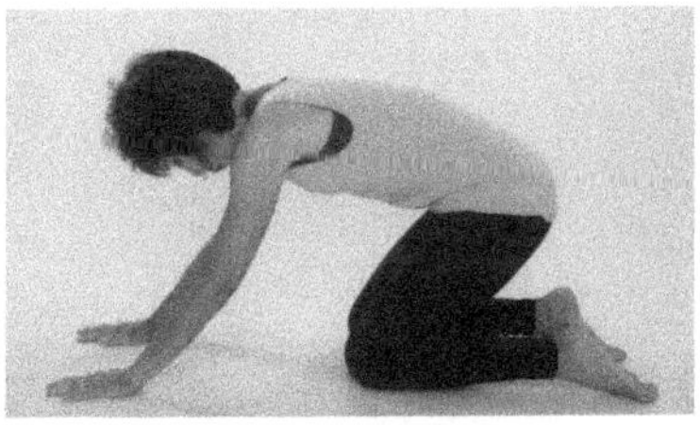

Photo 57

If you wish to work more intensely, try progressively increasing the holds to 3–4–5 seconds. Sustain a strong abdominal contraction during the suspension after each exhale. You might also try breaking the breath and movement into three parts—for example, exhaling back a third of the way, then two-thirds of the way, then fully into Child's Pose. Focus on refining the activation of the TVA with a more controlled contraction while emphasizing flexion of your lumbar spine. Maintain your JB chin tuck on the exhale.

(E) Baby Plank—Hover Position Knees Down (Photo 58)

In spite of the name, there is nothing "babyish" about this version of Plank. It is my personal favorite, because using the forearms as foundation provides stability through the shoulder girdle and there is absolutely no way to cheat. The TVA has to do the work! I use this adaptation with my therapeutic clients with low back pain and have come to trust it because, while it is intense and hard to hold, it is relatively safe and very effective. Maintain awareness of your ZOA throughout the Baby Plank series. Direct the engagement of the abdominals to synch with the exhale and narrow the rib cage for a complete core experience.

1. Lie prone on your belly.
2. Place your forearms on the floor, elbows a few inches forward of your shoulders.
3. Interlace your fingers.
4. Tuck your chin into a light JB and hold it there.
5. Keep your eye gaze towards the floor and maintain length at the back of your neck.
6. Lift your chest, contract your pecs and protract your shoulder blades (spread them apart).
7. Curl your toes under and keep your knees on the ground.
8. Engage your TVA and micro-lift your navel area, pelvis, and lower rib cage off the floor (see Photo 58).
9. Hover and hold position progressively for 2–6 seconds, as able.
10. Keep your ribs hugged in throughout the contraction.
11. Rest when fatigued. Then repeat, building reps as you are able.

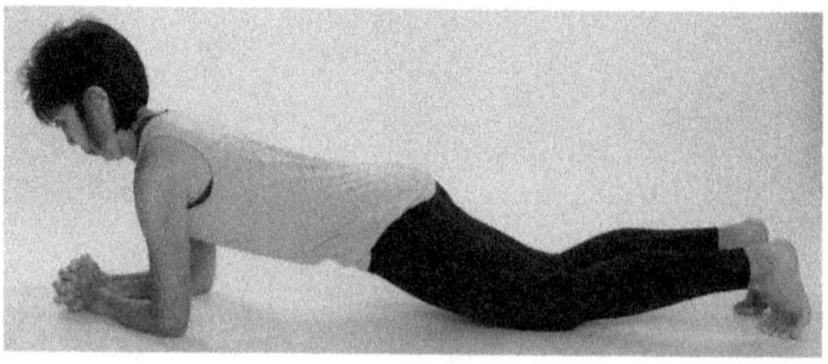

Photo 58

Note: If you are experiencing excessive pressure in your shoulder girdle tension, wriggle your toes back to create more length between your pelvis and your elbows. The further apart they are, the more effective the work of the abdominals and the less pressure on the upper back, shoulders, and arms.

The feeling created by this hover position is as if a bungee cord were drawing your ASIS (front bones of the pelvis) together and the triangular area between your hips and pubis are intensely lifting in, away from the floor. Once you have mastered this variation, try doing these Baby Planks lifting your upper thighs off the floor (knees are still down). Keep the pelvis low to the ground, maintaining passivity in your hamstrings and glutes. Your lower back should feel neutral as the work comes from the inside, not the back side.

Tip for success: Start the lift from your lower rib cage. This will initiate the action from the upper TVA and ZOA. Not only does this strengthen this area, but it offers far more support for the entire lumbar spine.

Baby Plank—Hover Position with Alternate Knee Lifts (Photos 59 and 60)

This variation is more intense, so take time to develop your TVA with the knees-down variations first. Notice that as the physical movement becomes more challenging, it is easy to generate bigger breaths. Practice keeping the breath silent and slow, calm and light, even while working your muscles strongly and building endurance.

1. Come up into Baby Plank with knees down (Photo 59).
2. Actively extend one leg at a time. Keep your toes curled and pressing into the floor. Lift your whole thigh and knee off the floor (Photo 60).
3. Hold for one second, then rest your knee down.
4. Alternately extend your right, then your left knee.
5. Stay in a low parallel hover with your body.
6. Maintain TVA activation and soft nose breathing throughout.
7. The key is to maintain horizontal stability through your pelvis as your knee lifts (no side-to-side wobble in your pelvis).
8. Rest down when fatigued.
9. Relax the breath.
10. Repeat 1–2 more sets as able.

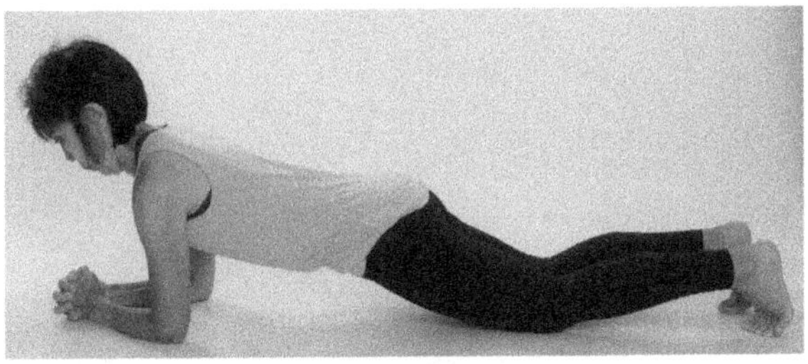

Photo 59

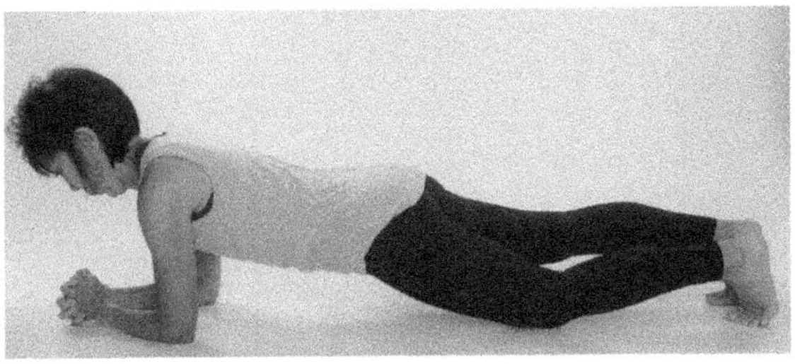

Photo 60

Variations: As strength builds, a slightly more intense version of this posture starts with your knees extended and requires alternately dropping one knee at a time to the floor. To build endurance, hold any of the plank positions static for longer periods of time, including both legs extended (see Photo 61).

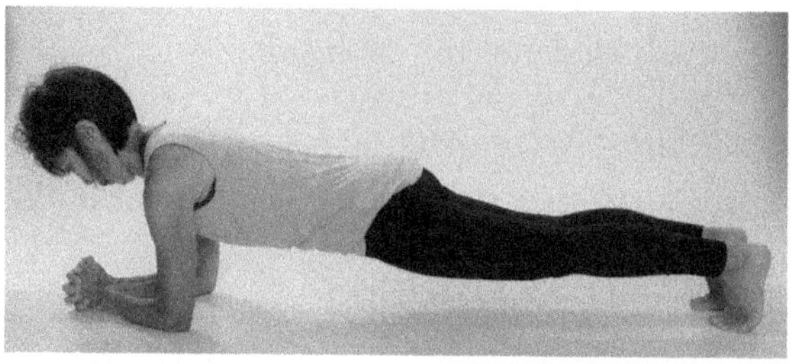

Photo 61

Counter Pose after Baby Plank with Child's Pose and Paint the Floor Undulation (Photo 62)

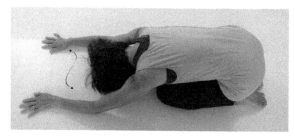

Photo 62

Charting the Practices to Develop the Transverse Abdominus (TVA)

Use the chart below to track your weekly progress with each of these TVA practices and describe the unique challenges you encounter. In the space provided below the chart, write your overall reflections of how these practices have informed your āsana practice and your svādhyāya of your breath patterns over the course of the month.

Developing the Transverse Abdominus Chart

Week 1

Type of Practice	Frequency	Reflections on Practice
Block Squeeze 2-Part Krama Exhale		
Knees to Chest 2-Part Krama Exhale		
Bridge with Block 2–3-Part Krama Exhale		
Wheel Pose 2-Part Krama Exhale		
Baby Plank—Knees Down		
Baby Plank—Knees Up		

Week 2

Type of Practice	Frequency	Reflections on Practice
Block Squeeze 2-Part Krama Exhale		
Knees to Chest 2-Part Krama Exhale		
Bridge with Block 2–3-Part Krama Exhale		
Wheel Pose 2-Part Krama Exhale		
Baby Plank—Knees Down		
Baby Plank—Knees Up		

Week 3

Type of Practice	Frequency	Reflections on Practice
Block Squeeze 2-Part Krama Exhale		
Knees to Chest 2-Part Krama Exhale		
Bridge with Block 2–3-Part Krama Exhale		
Wheel Pose 2-Part Krama Exhale		
Baby Plank—Knees Down		
Baby Plank—Knees Up		

Week 4

Type of Practice	Frequency	Reflections on Practice
Block Squeeze 2-Part Krama Exhale		
Knees to Chest 2-Part Krama Exhale		
Bridge with Block 2–3-Part Krama Exhale		
Wheel Pose 2-Part Krama Exhale		
Baby Plank—Knees Down		
Baby Plank—Knees Up		

PRACTICE 7.2: DEVELOPING YOUR PELVIC FLOOR SERIES

Working with the pelvic floor (PF) is more subtle, can be associated with sexual or bladder dysfunction, and can reignite past sexual trauma in some people. I therefore suggest you begin inner core work with the activation of the TVA and diaphragm prior to working with the PF. Working first with the TVA and Subtle and Core Breathing builds interoceptive awareness, which can translate into more self-confidence when exploring the recruitment of the PF.

That said, there are a few details to note when working with the PF. First of all, some people have hypertonic (tight or tense) PF muscles that chronically spasm. This can translate to pain in the lower back or in the sacrum and/or coccyx, and pain during sex, and can lead to incontinence. "Hypertonic" does not mean the muscles are strong, just ultra-tense. It is difficult to build strength in a muscle that is in spasm; resting tonus must be restored first. I have found that a combination—gentle contract, release, contract, release, explored slowly—is a more effective means to develop strength than contraction alone. This modality seems to "massage" the area into relaxation. It is a bit like getting your car out of a rut: You ease in reverse a little, then rock forward, reverse, then go forward. If you gun the engine unidirectionally, it digs the wheels deeper into the trench.

Kegel exercises, the standard approach to PF strengthening, are often taught in a gun-the-engine manner, meaning hard-fast contraction, hold at 100 percent for 10 seconds, then release. This is significantly different from the approach taken here. As you work, move slowly and cue yourself to consistently stay in the mid-range (somewhere between 10% and 85% effort), with as much emphasis given to the controlled release of the muscles as to their activation. Time the contraction of your pelvic floor muscles with the exhalation breath; inhale as you let them go.

(A) Bolster Straddle (Photo 63)

As the yoga teachings emphasize, we can only change what we are aware of. The initial (and often biggest) challenge with working with the PF is feeling the pelvic floor. I have found the Bolster Straddle a useful approach to take. Note the wording used to address male and female anatomical differences.

Kneeling from the floor:

- Straddle a firm yoga bolster (if available) in the vertical plane (lengthwise) or use three firm blankets stacked and rolled into a tight mound.
- The bolster is a means to create a sensory bio-feedback loop from the muscles of your pelvic floor to your brain—so you can feel more of what's happening "down there."
- **For female anatomy:** Lean slightly forward so your anal sphincter (and glutes) are less weighted. Firmly place your perineal floor (the area between your genitals and anus) onto the bolster, positioning yourself so the front end of your vaginal opening has firm contact with the support.
- Visualize the sling of the PF (use an anatomical diagram if that's helpful). There are muscles that run front to back; some run side to side; a third set creates a drawstring that gathers the layers and lifts them up towards the pubis. Visualize each of these layers and begin to activate them individually. Notice which ones you can recruit and which "flicker" into awareness and then are lost. This is all useful information. Once you have a sense of how to recruit the PF muscles, continue on with the Anemone Hand Pulses (see below) to refine your awareness and synch the pelvic floor action with the breath.

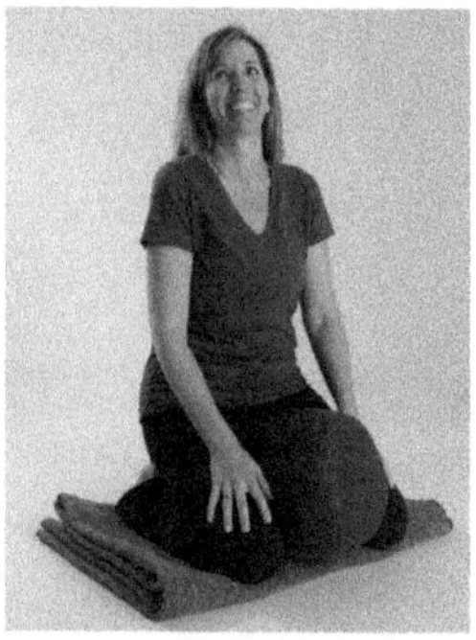

Photo 63

- **For male anatomy:** Place yourself on the bolster with care, so that your testes are comfy and you have contact with your perineal area, between your testes and anus. Imagine that you just stepped into a cold lake and feel the lift of your testes. Try drawing them in and up in greater or lesser degrees. Visualize the variations of lift options as per the sling description from above. Once you have a sense of how to recruit your PF muscles, continue on with the Anemone Hand Pulses (see below) to refine your awareness and synch the pelvic floor action with the breath.

Chair Variation with Blanket Roll (Photo 64)

The same process can be done while seated in a chair with a smaller blanket roll underneath your pelvic floor. This is a useful variation for those who cannot kneel or get down on the floor.

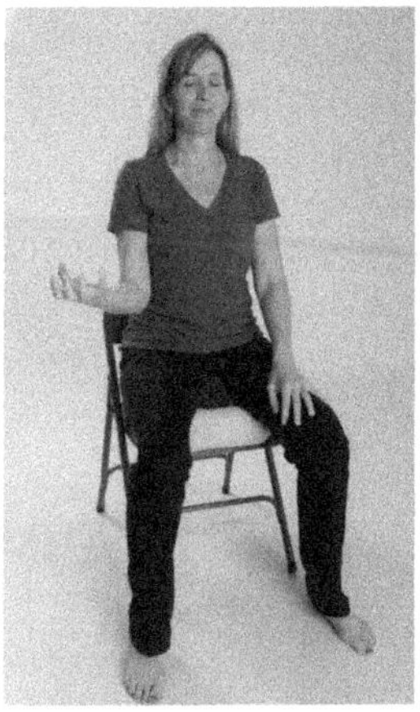

Photo 64

(B) Anemone Hand Pulses (Photos 65 and 66)

The image of an anemone conjures a soft and flowy undulation that mirrors the style of engagement we want to cultivate when working with the PF. Working with the PF can initially bring up doubt, as in "Do I really feel the muscles contracting? Am I releasing? Is it or is it not the pelvic floor?" Using your hand as a somatic cue to stimulate PF recruitment can help activate the muscles and synchronize their firing with the breath.

1. Turn one palm face up and hold it slightly up off your lap.
2. Make a tight fist with your hand and say to yourself, "100 percent contraction" (Photo 65).
3. Tighten your PF muscles to a similar degree.
4. Now open the palm of your hand fully—free of contraction. Say to yourself, "0 percent contraction" (Photo 66).
5. Relax your PF muscles as completely as you can to match your hand position.
6. Now that you have the parameters, play the middle ground…
7. Take your hand into a 20 percent contraction and follow with your PF, contracting 20 percent.
8. Relax your hand and PF by 5 percent, so you're at 15% contraction.
9. Then bump up the contraction to 46.5 percent.[2]
10. Cue your PF to follow the contraction or release of your hand.
11. Relax by 12.2 percent.
12. Continue to play Follow the Leader with your PF in this way, exploring the in-between places and spaces for contraction and release.

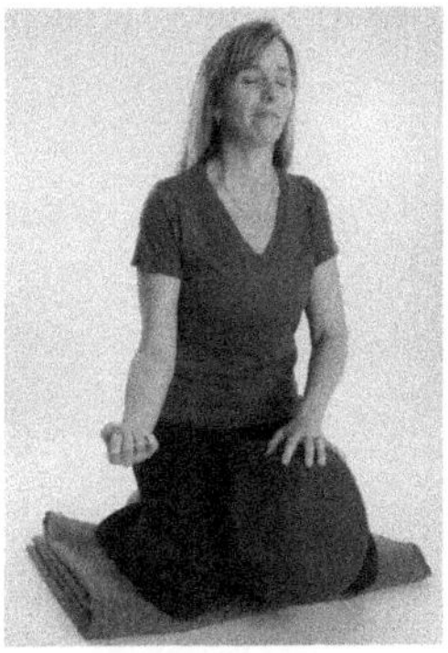

Photo 65

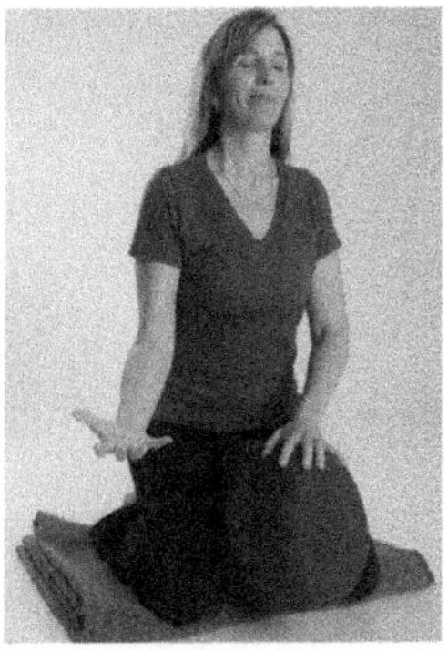

Photo 66

You can even work in a krama fashion: Exhale partially and contract 7.7 percent. Then exhale a little more and contract another 3 percent. Then exhale a little more and contract 9.3 percent. Then, inhale and release 17.5 percent. Breath size will vary according to how large or small the krama movement.

Reminder: In the interest of establishing the recruitment of your PF to synch with your breath, consistently link your exhalation with the action of contraction, and your inhalation with conscious release. Sip your breath, rather than gulp it. Keep your in-breath soft and light. Each movement and the accompanying breath mirror each other.

As you become more aware of and proficient at activating the PF muscles, especially the drawstring lift, you'll automatically feel the engagement of your lower TVA recruiting as well. This is a sign of your growing proprioceptive awareness of the fascial connections. Building on this awareness, begin to follow the kinetic chain up from your lower to upper TVA, to your diaphragm, and back down again, working in a krama style. I've heard this referred to metaphorically as the "Elevator Technique" (i.e. lift to the first "floor," then the third, drop down to the second, down into the basement...). Work with any metaphors and visualizations that help you to connect to the PF muscles and feel comfortable with both their recruitment and release.

(C) Dynamic Butterfly Pose—Supta Baddhakonasana (Photos 67–70)

To take the PF action to the next level, try working with Dynamic Butterfly Pose, either from a supine position or seated in a chair. Both are extremely valuable and each has a unique impact on the spine and pelvic girdle. When working on a chair, start with the Seated Mountain Pose position. You may need to sit slightly forward on the chair, so your hips can open freely (Photo 67). The outside edges of your feet press firmly on the floor. Feel as if you are lifting your sit-bones slightly off the chair, as if you are about to launch, so your glutes and hamstrings are activated as well. Check in with your rib cage and set it in neutral. Maintain a neutral lumbar curve, as it provides more support for your lower back.

1. Bring the soles of your feet together and open (abduct) your hips, taking your thighs apart (Photo 68).
2. This position correlates with the PF at 0 percent recruitment (thighs together and touching reflects 100 percent contraction).
3. Work your PF as described above in the Anemone Hand Pulses. Coordinate the closing (adduction) and opening (abduction) of your thighs in time with the PF contraction and release.
4. As you exhale, begin to adduct your thighs and gently contract your PF.
5. As you inhale, begin to abduct your thighs and gently release your PF.

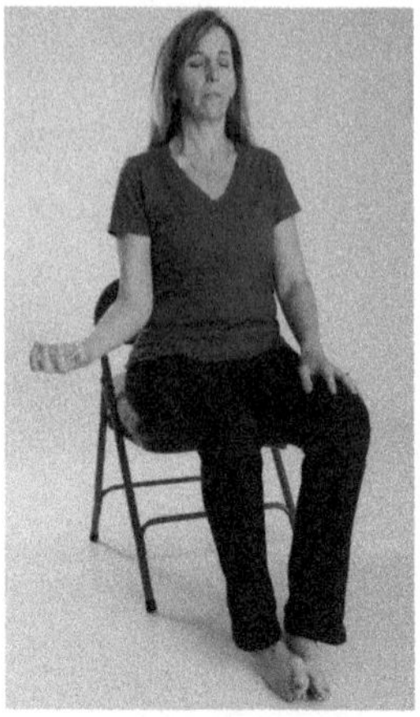

Photo 67
Chair Variation

6. Play the middle ground: Exhale and adduct your thighs and zip up your PF a percentage of the way. Inhale and abduct your thighs a percentage of the way, relaxing your PF accordingly.
7. It is easiest to start with pre-determined amounts, such as moving halfway open/closed, two-thirds of the way open/closed, three-quarters of the way open/closed (Photo 69).
8. Once you feel confident with this action, play with the in-between places, using micro-movements to finely attune your awareness.
9. When fatigued, you may feel your thighs begin to shake or you may lose the ability to actively recruit your PF muscles. Place your feet on the floor. Rest. Undulate your neck and shoulders to release any accrued tension. Then repeat another set of the Dynamic Butterfly.

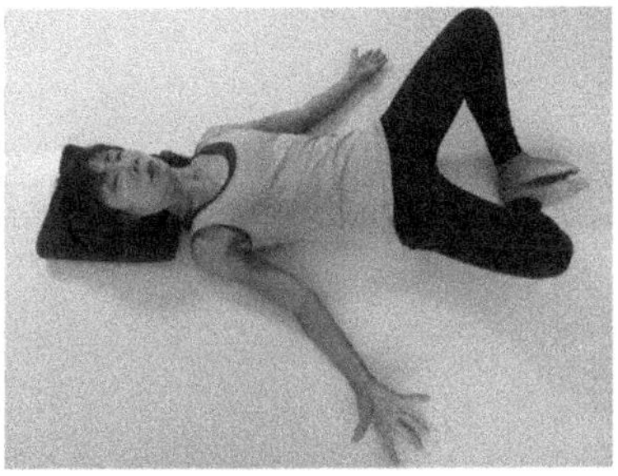

Photo 68

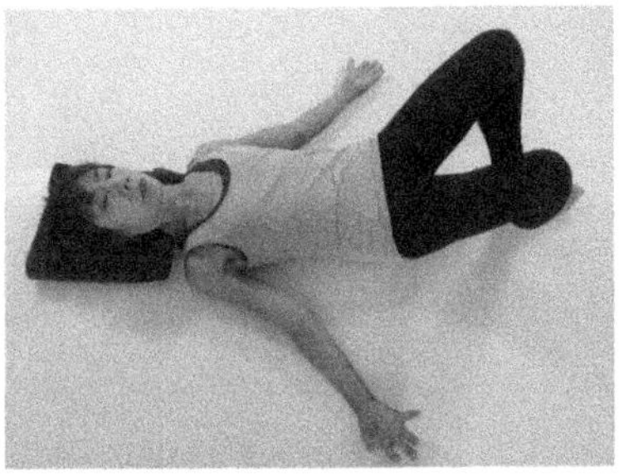

Photo 69

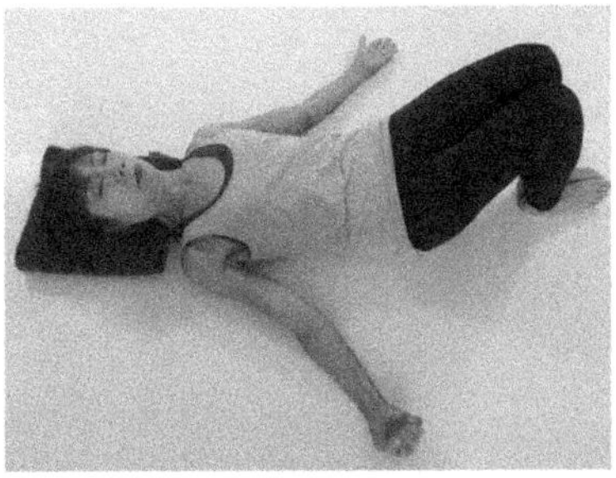

Photo 70

Movement in this posture creates a wonderful link from the adductor complex, through the PF, and up into the TVA and abdominals. It is particularly useful to continue that DFL kinetic chain up through the spine, to the ribs, mid-back, and into the cervical alignment by creating a slight jālandhara bandha set to the chin. Working with tiny micro-movements (a half-inch in, half-inch out) can help you identify areas of low proprioceptive awareness, or places that you identify are weak or tight along the way. Note for practitioners who are very flexible in hip abduction: I recommend limiting your range to approximately three-quarters of the way open, particularly in the supine position. This will avert the possibility of hanging in the hip joints and over-stretching the ligaments.

Charting the Practices to Develop the Pelvic Floor

Use the chart below to track your weekly progress with each of these PF practices and describe the unique challenges you encounter. In the space provided below the chart, write your overall reflections of how these practices have informed your āsana practice and your svādhyāya of your breath patterns over the course of the month.

Developing the Pelvic Floor Chart

Week 1

Type of Practice	Frequency	Reflections on Practice
Bolster Straddle		
Anemone Hand Pulses		
Dynamic Butterfly		

Week 2

Type of Practice	Frequency	Reflections on Practice
Bolster Straddle		
Anemone Hand Pulses		
Dynamic Butterfly		

Week 3

Type of Practice	Frequency	Reflections on Practice
Bolster Straddle		
Anemone Hand Pulses		
Dynamic Butterfly		

Week 4

Type of Practice	Frequency	Reflections on Practice
Bolster Straddle		
Anemone Hand Pulses		
Dynamic Butterfly		

Note: The term *core* is most frequently associated with recruitment of the deep abdominal and pelvic floor muscles. I have used the terms *mid-back core* and *neck core* as complements to the abdominal core, in order to link the pelvis, mid-torso, and neck in a stabilizing fashion. These additional "cores" will be described fully in the practices below. The combined and consistent recruitment of the "cores" assists both functional movement and functional breathing.

PRACTICE 7.3: DEVELOPING THE MID-BACK CORE SERIES

To fully integrate diaphragmatic action and increase the ZOA, we need to give equal attention to the action both above and below the diaphragm. Mobilization, strength, and proper positioning of the mid-back, ribs, and shoulder girdle play a significant role in resolving breathing pattern disorders, such as chest and paradoxical breathing. While the undulations described in Chapter 6 are very useful for releasing tension and "unhooking" the upper shoulder girdle from the act of breathing, learning how to anchor the scapula and stabilize what I call the "mid-back core" (MBC) is of equal importance.

The MBC comprises the serratus anterior, the lower portion of the rhomboids, the rotator cuff muscles, and the lower traps. Together they work synergistically to establish cohesive action of the shoulder blades. This prevents "chest droop" and the tendency to collapse the front of the rib cage down into the belly. That said, "rib-jutters" beware! Working with the MBC can feel like an invitation to slide into the old hyperextension saṃskāra. Maintain a gentle "knitting" or drawing inward of the lower rib cage while working the MBC. This will illuminate tight areas in the pecs, the iliopsoas, the lats, or even the neck that have been bypassed through habituation of the forward displacement of the rib cage.

(A) Wide V/Narrow V with PF and TVA Engagement from Supine Position (Photos 71 and 72 Correct, Photos 73 and 74 Incorrect)

The Vs referenced in the title of this exercise refer to the angle of the arms. Narrow Vs reflect a drawing in of the shoulder blades (retraction), thus narrowing the space between the upper arm and the rib cage. Wide Vs press the shoulder blades apart (protraction) and widen the space between the arms and the torso. Note: The V-shape angle of the elbow through the forearm remains the same. The photos below demonstrate the correct (Photos 71 and 72) and incorrect (Photos 73 and 74) action of the shoulder blades for this exercise. The actual pose is done supine, with the knees and elbows bent, starting with Core Breathing.

1. Begin supine with Core Breathing.
2. Insert a block between your mid-thighs (not between or pressing on your knees).
3. Engage a light DFL awareness with your adductors.
4. Set your upper arm bones in external rotation (see Photo 54).
5. Do some Scapular Swirls and Passing Notes to wake up your shoulder blades.
6. Bend your elbows and angle your arms so your thumb tips touch down to the floor (Photo 71).
7. Adjust the angle to make this possible at a degree that keeps the tops of your shoulders passive, your breath light, and your rib cage set in neutral.
8. Feel free to place a small towel or blanket under your neck and head to help pacify your neck, jaw, and upper traps.
9. On the inhale, protract your shoulder blades and widen the angle between your upper arms and your spine (Photo 72).
10. On the exhale, retract your shoulder blades and narrow the angle between your upper arms and your spine (Photo 71).
11. Notice that it is possible to move your elbows/arms in and out and not mobilize your shoulder blades. How is it different to initiate movement from your scapula rather than your elbows?
12. Notice if your ribs "pop up" when your shoulder blades draw in. How do you interpret this action?
13. Notice if your lumbar area hyperextends with the narrow Vs. How do you interpret this action?
14. Notice if your chin lifts, or your shoulders cup forward or tense when your blades retract. How do you interpret this action? How can you pacify these areas and work your mid-back in isolation?

15. Regularly intersperse undulations such as Paint the Floor, Doodle, or Passing Notes to release tension in your upper back and neck as you work with the Vs.
16. Do another rep of Vs in and out. Remember to always work *slow*, *slow*, *slow*, and time the movement with the breath.
17. Return to Core Breathing and notice the effect of the process.

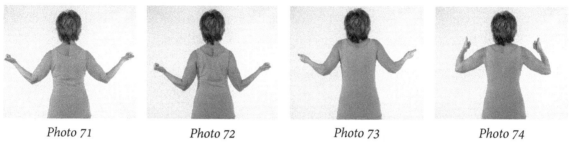

Photo 71

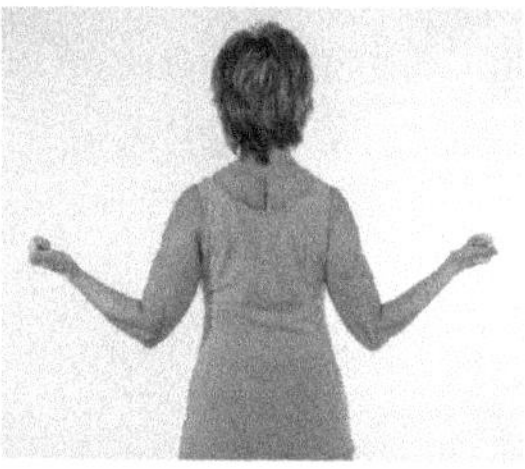

Photo 72

Correct Action

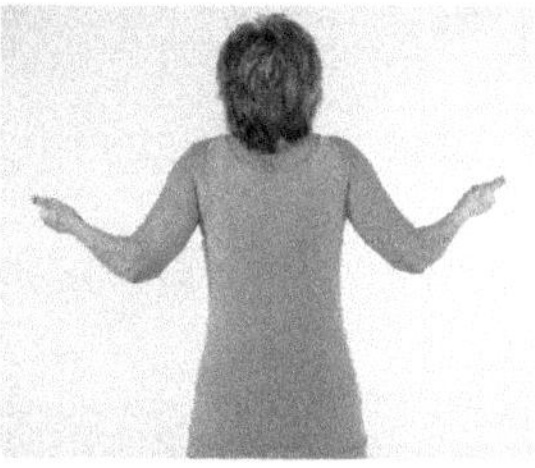

Photo 73

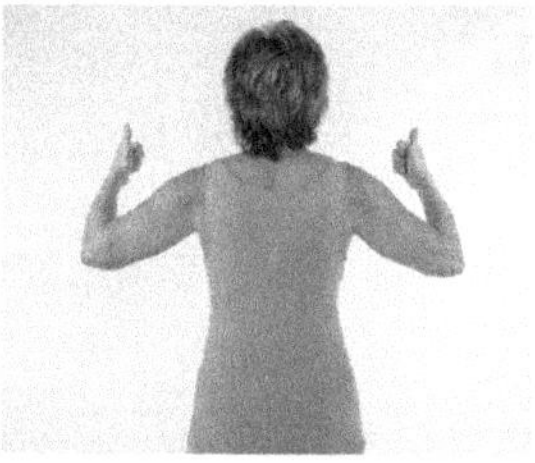

Photo 74

Incorrect Action

(B) Linking It Together (Photos 75–77)

To weave together the kinetic chain of the abdominal core and mid-back core with the breath, let's start from the base and work through to the top, linking the PF, TVA, and a light jālandhara bandha (JB; neck core engagement) with the recruitment of the mid-back.

1. Begin supine with Core Breathing.
2. Insert a block between your mid-thighs (not between or pressing on your knees).
3. Engage a light DFL awareness with your adductors.
4. Set your upper body as above for Wide V/Narrow Vs, with arms set in external rotation.
5. Inhale and set your chin in slightly, creating a gentle jālandhara bandha.
6. As you exhale, engage your pelvic floor muscles lightly and contract your TVA to your lower ribs.
7. Hold the abdominal core contraction and draw the shoulder blades into a narrow V.
8. On the next inhale, release your TVA from your rib cage to your pubis, and protract your scapula in a wide V.
9. Repeat another 4–6 rounds of Vs with core engagement, cueing yourself as you breathe in and out.
10. As much as possible, isolate your mid-body, focusing on mini-movement of the diaphragm and shoulder blades. Maintain consistent stabilization through your PF, TVA, and neck.

11. Notice if your chin lifts or juts forward.

12. Notice if your block squeeze lightens or tightens.

13. Notice if your lumbar arches more or less in response to the movement.

14. Notice the challenge for you in keeping the core movement integrated and flowing with the breath.

15. Intersperse any of the undulations that help release and relax the neck and shoulders between reps. Vs with core engagement can be also performed in Butterfly Pose, Bridge Pose (Photos 75 and 76), Standing/Seated Mountain Pose, Chair Pose, or Warrior 1 (Photo 77) among others. Each position offers a different way of increasing awareness of the kinetic chain and its own unique challenge.

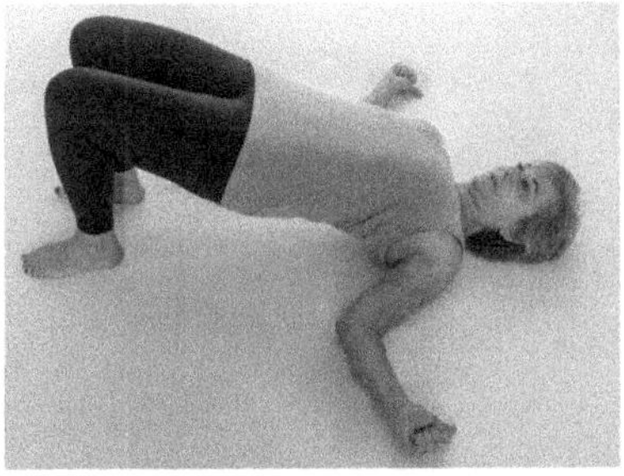

Photo 75

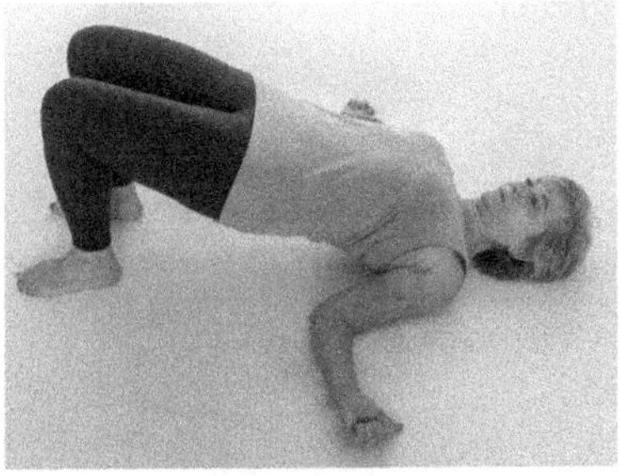

Photo 76

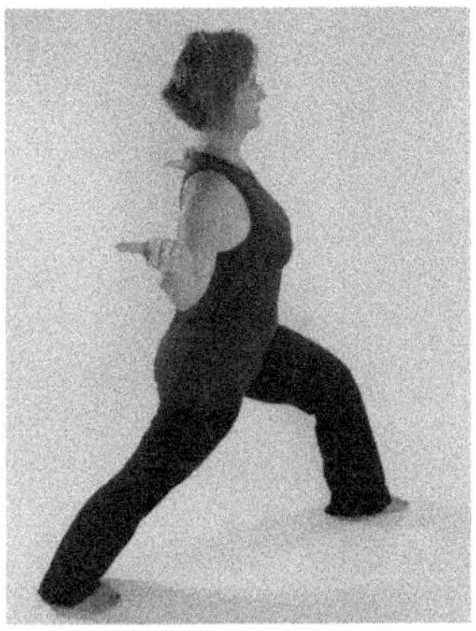

Photo 77

(C) Shalambhāsana (Locust Pose) (Photos 78–80)

This is another position that works well with the Vs. As it requires more strength, I tend to be cautious with people who are more vulnerable in the lower back or cervical areas when working with this particular variation. It may be weeks or even months before I introduce it.

Working with the core muscles in prone backbends integrates a feeling similar to Baby Plank through the TVA. Maintaining upper-back extension and the JB tuck of the chin strengthens the whole body. Diaphragmatic Hugs can be added to this series for a full-on body-breath workout!

1. Lie prone (face down) and place a block between your calves.

2. Engage a light DFL awareness with your calf muscles.

3. Bend your elbows into wide Vs and tip the thumbs up in a "hitchhiking" position (Photo 78).

4. Tip your elbows low and inward towards your lower ribs, activating your MBC while creating a feeling of neutrality along your upper traps.

5. On the exhale, squeeze the block, zip up your PF and TVA.

6. On the inhale, maintain your core engagement below and lift your chest, head, and forearms.
7. Hold your eye gaze down towards the floor and sustain a gentle JB in the neck.
8. Remain lifted, and on the exhale, retract your scapula, bringing your elbows in closer to your rib cage while maintaining a strong Diaphragmatic Hug (Photo 79).
9. Hold 3–4 seconds.
10. Remain lifted, and on the inhale, expand your rib cage laterally, protract your scapula, and fan your upper arms out slightly—an inch or two farther from your torso (Photo 80).
11. Remain lifted, and on the exhale, retract your scapula once again. Draw your arms in. Keep your abdominal core engaged.
12. Hold for 3–4 seconds.
13. Rest down and relax.
14. Pause and breathe gently, then repeat the sequence.
15. As strength builds, stay up and work in sets of 3–6 breaths at a time.

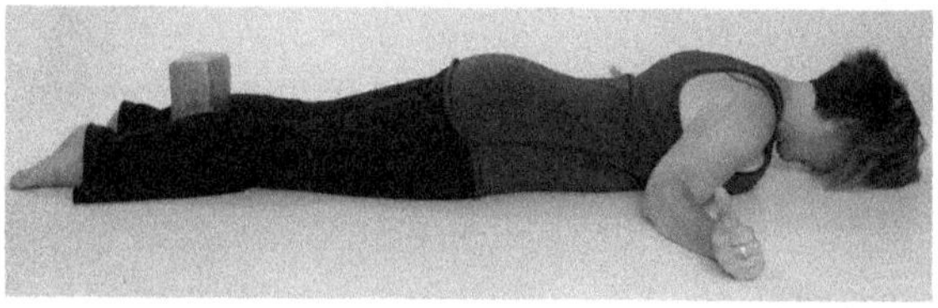

Photo 78

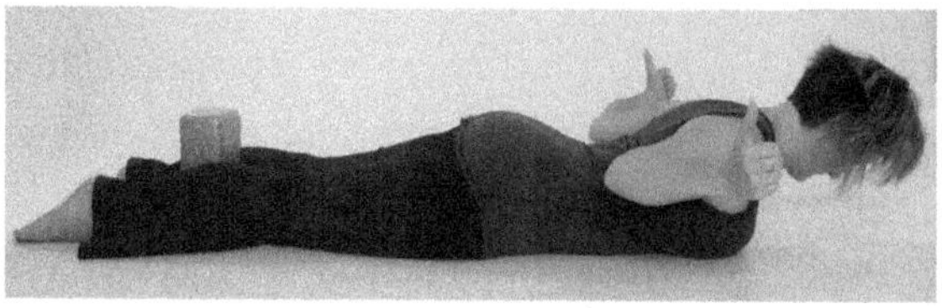

Photo 79

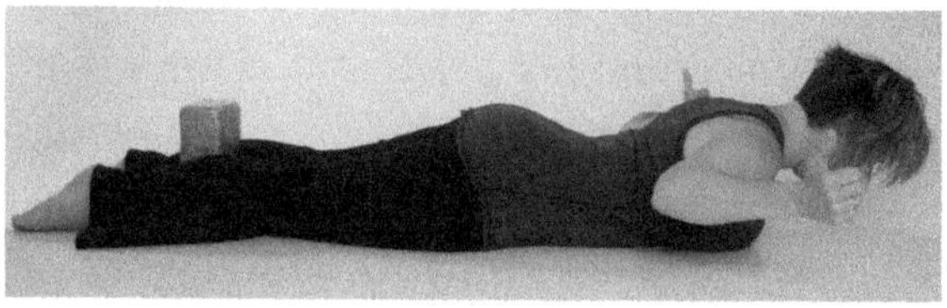

Photo 80

Note: In the back extension, angle the arms so the thumbs are higher than the elbows at all times. Notice that when elbows lift and the thumbs drop towards the floor, the shoulders will cup forward into internal rotation. This disengages the MBC. Instead, prioritize the proper set of the blades over the height of the lift of the chest or limbs. Even lifting the chest and arms an inch with proper positioning of the arms is beneficial.

Counter Pose Options for Shalambhāsana (Locust Pose): Wheel Pose, Child's Pose, Paint the Floor, and Scapular Swirls as Needed

Charting the Practices to Develop the Mid-Back Core

Use the chart below to track your weekly progress with each of these MBC practices and describe the unique challenges you encounter. In the space provided below the chart, write your overall reflections of how these practices have informed your āsana practice and your svādhyāya of your breath patterns over the course of the month.

Developing the Mid-Back Core Chart

Week 1

Type of Practice	Frequency	Reflections on Practice
Wide V/Narrow V—Supine		
Linking MBC with PF, TVA and JB in āsana		
Shalambhāsana with Wide V/ Narrow V		

Week 2

Type of Practice	Frequency	Reflections on Practice
Wide V/Narrow V—Supine		
Linking MBC with PF, TVA and JB in āsana		
Shalambhāsana with Wide V/ Narrow V		

Week 3

Type of Practice	Frequency	Reflections on Practice
Wide V/Narrow V—Supine		
Linking MBC with PF, TVA and JB in āsana		
Shalambhāsana with Wide V/ Narrow V		

Week 4

Type of Practice	Frequency	Reflections on Practice
Wide V/Narrow V—Supine		
Linking MBC with PF, TVA and JB in āsana		
Shalambhāsana with Wide V/ Narrow V		

PRACTICE 7.4: DEVELOPING THE NECK CORE SERIES

Headstand and prāṇāyāma share a similar saga in that during the era from which they evolved, the posture, stamina, and quality of life required of the practitioners were a good match for the challenge of these practices. Headstand essentially takes the DFL and puts it in reverse relative to gravity. It is a pose that requires a solid core line, especially the mid-back and neck core. The condition of the neck and shoulder girdle of the average yoga practitioner these days provides a less than adequate foundation for the strength and integration required for a healthy headstand practice. That said, one does not develop a strong neck core without doing strength work. The following are my top favorite and accessible neck strengtheners that I use routinely in my therapeutic practice. Integration of the abdominal core and MBC work from the exercises above is a critical ingredient to ensuring that the neck position is well supported by the whole DFL.

(A) Baby Fish 1-2-3-3-2-1 (Photos 81-83)

This position is sequenced in a stepped fashion, when transitioning into and out of the posture to ensure the neck is never left hanging. Position the flat of the tongue up into the roof of the mouth and keep it there throughout the practice.

1. Begin supine with Core Breathing.
2. Engage a light DFL awareness from your inner arches to your adductors and abdominal core.
3. Bend your elbows and set them firmly in next to your rib cage. Press the backs of your upper arms into the floor, to create a strong brace of support for your neck.
4. Set your forearms parallel to one another, perpendicular to the floor.
5. Make a light fist with your hands (Photo 81).
6. Press your elbows down into the floor and lift your chest and upper back.
7. Engage your MBC strongly. Draw your scapulae in away from the floor. Lift your upper sternum more than your lower ribs to avoid a big forward jut of your rib cage. Your upper back and scapula lift up away from the floor. Buttocks stay on the floor (Photo 82).
8. Press the back of your head into the floor and lift your chin up. Your neck will extend as you roll your head towards your crown (Photo 83).
9. Hold for 2–3 breaths.

To come out of Baby Fish, reverse the action as follows:

10. Start by tucking your chin to release your neck (Photo 82).
11. Relax your upper back, letting it come to rest on the floor again (Photo 81).
12. Release the strong downward thrust of the upper arms, relaxing the brace of support.

13. Take a resting breath or two and then repeat the process 1–2–3–3–2–1. Progressively stay for more breath cycles as able.
14. Follow Baby Fish pose with the undulations that feel most relaxing to you.

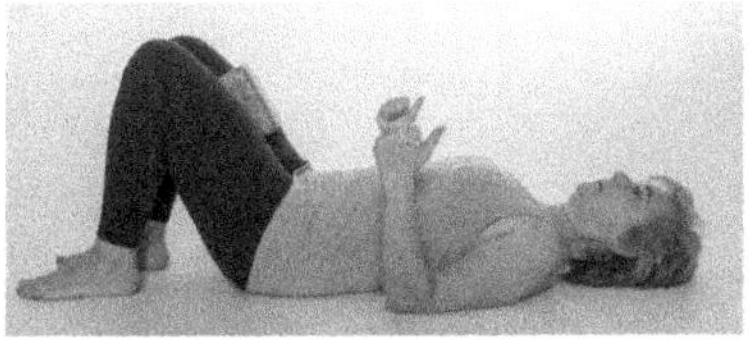
Photo 81

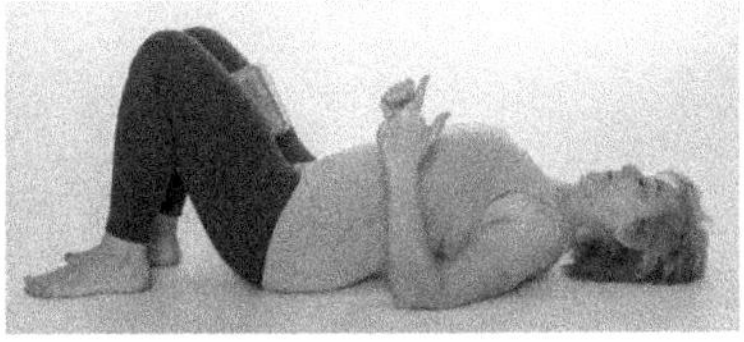
Photo 82

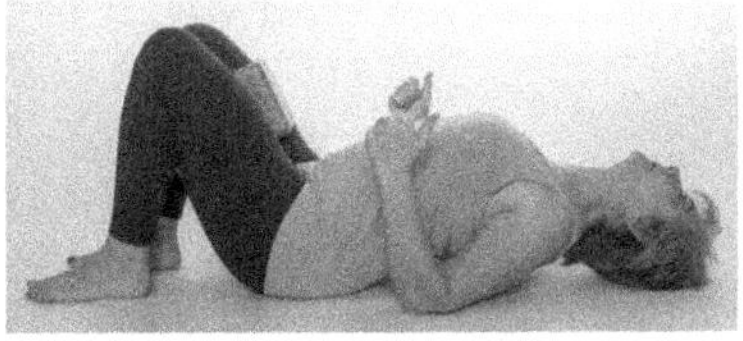
Photo 83

Note: To avoid compressing your neck, bring as much PF, TVA, and ZOA awareness into this process as possible, so your neck isn't hanging in hyperextension without support. To avoid compressing the back of your neck, visualize a small grapefruit positioned at the base of your skull and imagine draping your head up and over it, rather than jamming your head back as far as possible.

(B) Masthead (Photos 84–87)

Masthead is done from a standing position at a wall. For some people it is an easier starting point than Baby Fish. For others it works better as a second option. Due to the straight-legged position and diagonal orientation with the wall, it is tempting to sag into the lumbar area. Avoid this, as it will droop the chest and leave the neck without proper support. That said, Masthead is a favorite among my therapeutic students. They love the feeling of integration and connection they experience through the back of their body and the sense that their neck is effortlessly set in proper alignment with their shoulders.

1. Stand in Mountain Pose at the wall.
2. Place the back of your head on the wall and center it.
3. Step your heels about 1.5 feet (45 cm) away from the wall.
4. Insert a block between your mid-thighs (not between or pressing on your knees) (Photo 84).
5. Engage a light DFL awareness with your adductors.
6. Exhale—squeeze the block and zip up your abdominals from the bottom to the top.
7. Check in with your ribs and be sure they are set in neutral.
8. With the inhale lift your buttocks off the wall.
9. Open your arms approximately 30 degrees out from your body. Lift your chest and sternum without jutting the ribs (Photo 85).

10. Keep your chin in neutral, so your neck is neither flexed nor hyperextended.
11. Hold for 2–4 breaths.
12. To come out of the pose, step one foot back and press yourself forward into Mountain Pose away from the wall (Photo 86).
13. Pause and feel (Photo 87).
14. Repeat 2–3 times as comfortable.

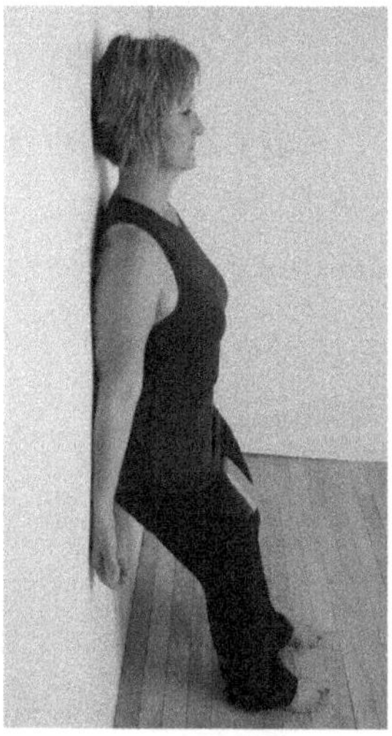

Photo 84

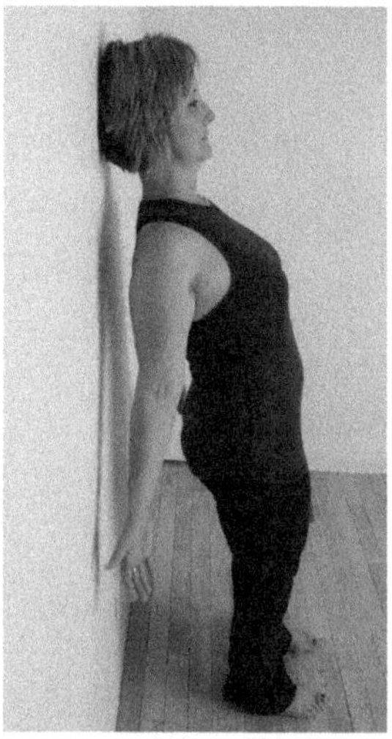

Photo 85

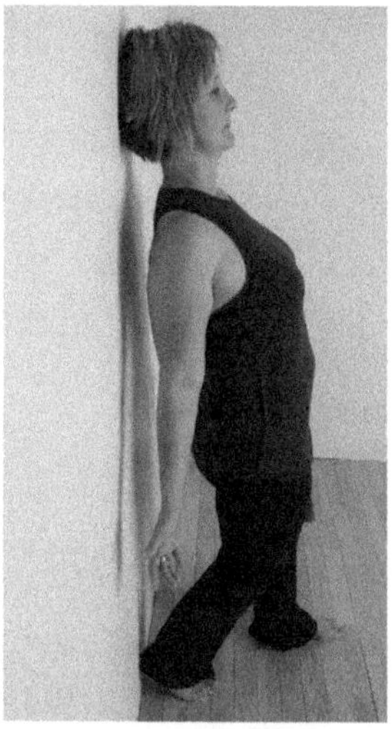

Photo 86

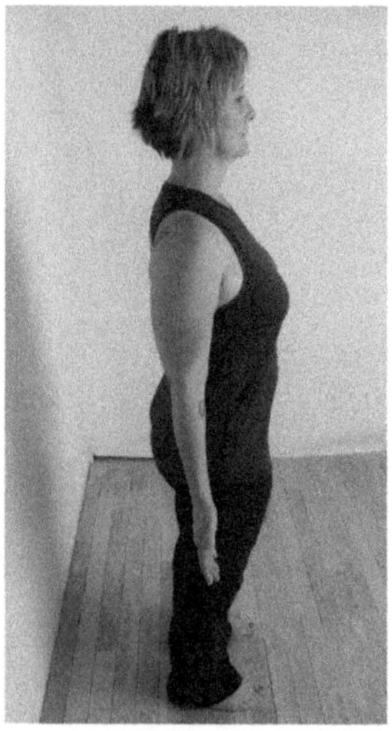

Photo 87

Counter Pose for Masthead: Uttanāsana (Standing Forward Fold) with Passing Notes and Rapunzel Undulations (Photo 88)

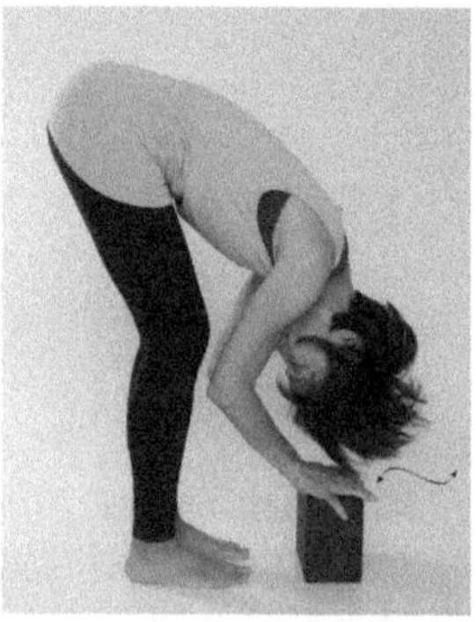

Photo 88

(C) Neck Core Lifts (Photos 91 and 92 Correct, Photos 93 and 94 Incorrect)

This exercise is useful for identifying the weak links of the neck core and working isometrically to strengthen it. The key is to vertically lift the head rather than flex the neck, and to honor the potency of the micro-movement and slow engagement of the muscles. The lift is tiny, a hair's breadth away from the floor.

1. Begin supine with Core Breathing.
2. Insert a block between your mid-thighs (not between or pressing on your knees).
3. Engage a light DFL awareness with your adductors.
4. Extend your index and middle fingers of both hands. Curl your thumb, ring finger, and pinky into your palm (Photo 89).
5. Place the tips of your index and middle fingers on either side of the very base of the skull, around C1 (Photo 90).
6. Rest your elbows on the floor or use blankets for comfort (Photo 90).
7. Draw your chin in to a gentle JB.
8. From the spot where the fingertips are placed, lift your head slightly as you exhale—maybe half an inch (1 cm) off the floor. Use your upper front neck muscles to create the lift, not your hands (Photo 92).
9. Hold for 1–2 seconds.
10. Inhale and relax down. Repeat the movement with that same cueing position of the hands 1–2 more times.
11. Your hands act merely as a point of reference, they do not assist in the lift of the head. The muscles of your neck core are entirely responsible for the action. Your neck should not flex (Photo 93) or extend (Photo 94). The movement is a straight vertical lift with JB held firmly in place.
12. Next, position your fingertips at the junction of C1–C2. Repeat the lifting process twice, then try moving them down to C2–C3, etc. Progress until you reach the base of your neck or experience fatigue and are unable to lift your head while firmly maintaining JB.
13. Notice how the experience changes as you progressively work lower down on your cervical spine.

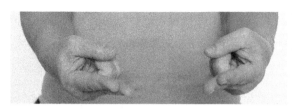

Photo 89

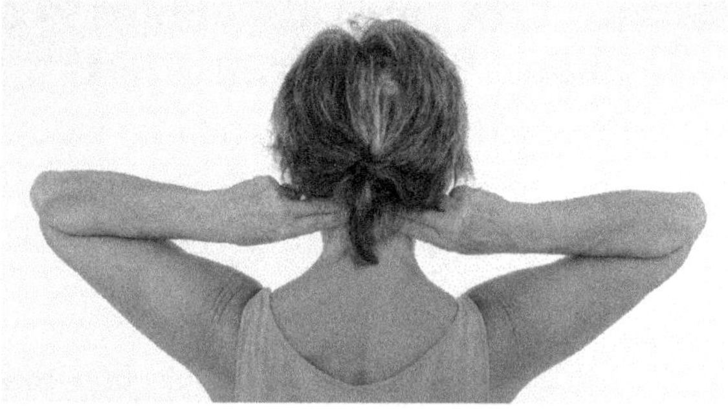

Photo 90

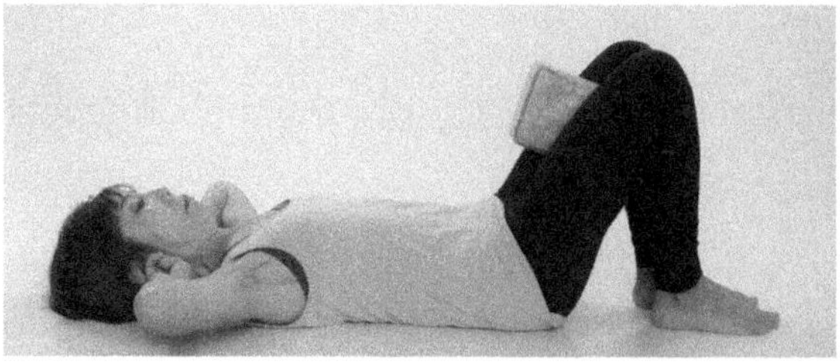

Photo 91

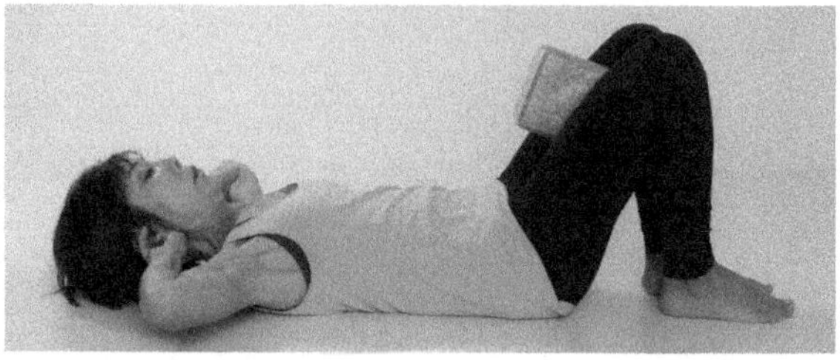

Photo 92

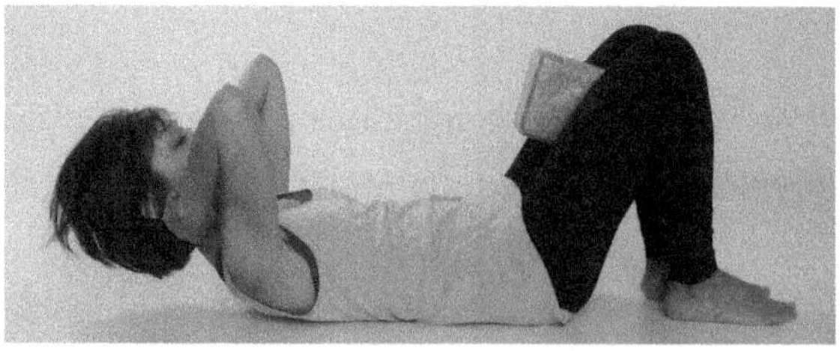

Photo 93

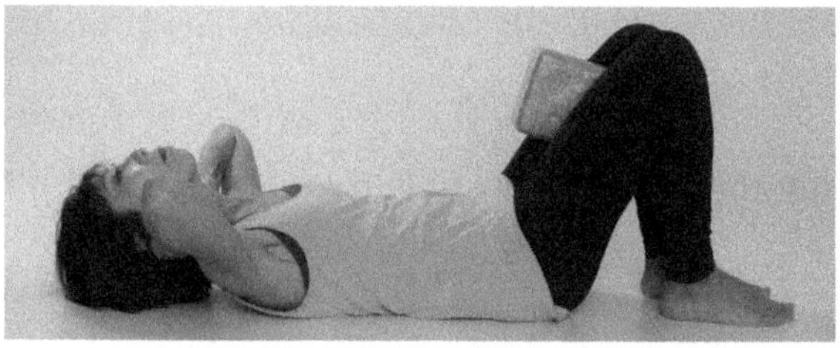

Photo 94

Most people find that as the point of the lift moves further away from the occiput (away from the base of the skull and towards the base of the neck), the action becomes more tiring and difficult to engage. It may take a number of weeks of regular practice before one can move much beyond C2 or C3. Build slowly until you are able to lift and hold comfortably through C7. Always stop and rest (and undulate) when you are fatigued.

Signs of compensation:

- The neck flexes in and the head lifts higher than half an inch (1 cm). This indicates recruitment of other muscles, not just the neck core (Photo 93).
- Hyperextension of the neck, inability to sustain the JB action with the chin tuck (Photo 94).
- The arms or hands are holding the weight of the head.

(D) Chair Pose at the Wall (Photos 95–99)

This posture is a wonderful way to integrate all three cores safely and in synchronization with the breath.

1. Stand with your back against a wall.
2. Step your heels out your thighs' length from the wall. Set your feet and legs parallel to one another.
3. Bend your knees in a soft squat.
4. Insert a block between your mid-thighs (not between or pressing on your knees).
5. Engage a light DFL awareness with your adductors.
6. Externally rotate your arms and set your shoulders so the wings of your shoulder blades retract (Photo 95).
7. Notice the positioning of the pelvis and be sure to create a neutral curve, not flattened (Photo 96) or excessively arched (Photo 97).
8. Bend your elbows so your forearms rest on the wall, with the palms facing forward.
9. If it is comfortable for your neck, rest your head on the wall while creating a light JB tuck of your chin.
10. If it strains your neck to rest your head on the wall, then create a light JB tuck of your chin and simply move the back of your head *towards* the wall without forcing contact.
11. Turn your palms so that the tips of your thumbs touch the wall. Prepare your shoulder blades for Narrow and Wide Vs.
12. Exhale and squeeze the block, gently contracting your core muscles from your PF to your TVA.
13. Simultaneously, draw in at your ZOA and retract your shoulder blades into a narrow V (Photo 98). This engages your MBC.
14. Keep your chin tucked and hold 2–4 seconds.
15. On the inhale, press down through your legs and slide your pelvis up the wall two to three inches, while widening the V of your arms, protracting your scapula (Photo 99). Check for rib-jut.
16. On the exhale, slide your pelvis down, engage your abdominals and retract your scapula into Narrow Vs.
17. Repeat this movement 3–5 times or until fatigued.
18. Keep your jaw and upper traps relaxed.

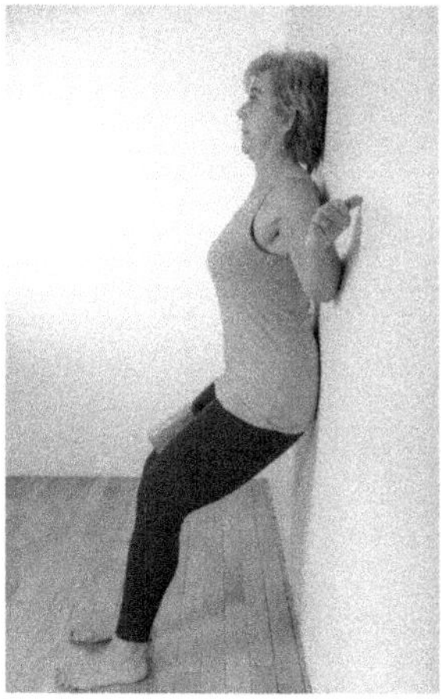

Photo 95 Correct Neutral Lumbar Curve

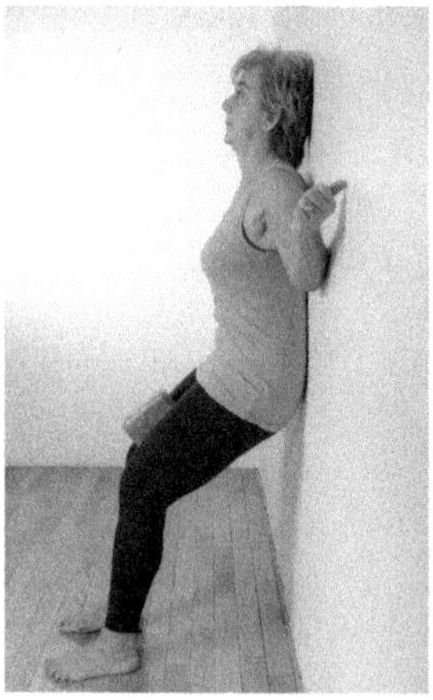

Photo 96 Lumbar Flattened

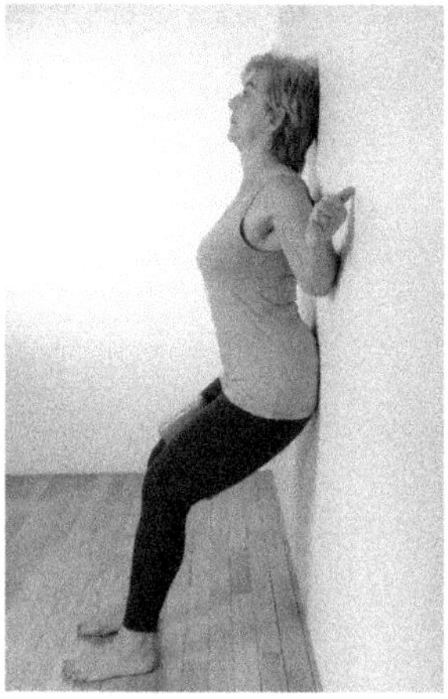

Photo 97 Lumbar Excessively Arched

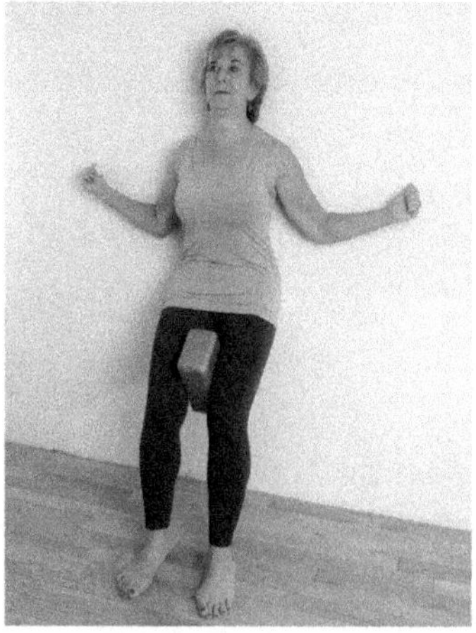

Photo 98 Narrow V Position in Chair Pose

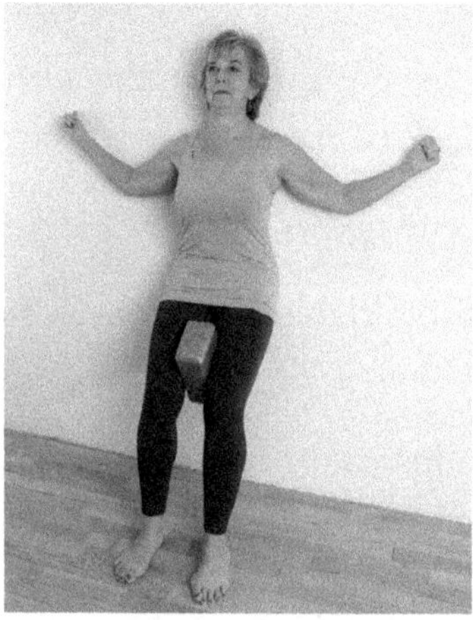

Photo 99 Wide V Position in Chair Pose

Use undulations including the Forward Bend and Rapunzel between sets or repetitions to avoid accumulating tension in your neck, jaw, and upper body. Consistently keep your breath light and low in the body. As with all of these exercises, maintain the proper positioning of your tongue, pressing to the roof of your mouth (upper palate). This facilitates better diaphragmatic action and engagement of the neck core.

Charting the Practices for Developing the Neck Core

Use the chart below to track your weekly progress with each of these Neck Core practices and describe the unique challenges you encounter. In the space provided below the chart, write your overall reflections of how these practices have informed your āsana practice and your svādhyāya of your breath patterns over the course of the month.

Developing the Neck Core Chart

Week 1

Type of Practice	Frequency	Reflections on Practice
Baby Fish 1–2–3–3–2–1		
Masthead		
Neck Core Lifts		
Integrated Core Work in Chair at Wall		

Week 2

Type of Practice	Frequency	Reflections on Practice
Baby Fish 1–2–3–3–2–1		
Masthead		
Neck Core Lifts		
Integrated Core Work in Chair at Wall		

Week 3

Type of Practice	Frequency	Reflections on Practice
Baby Fish 1–2–3–3–2–1		
Masthead		
Neck Core Lifts		
Integrated Core Work in Chair at Wall		

Week 4

Type of Practice	Frequency	Reflections on Practice
Baby Fish 1–2–3–3–2–1		
Masthead		
Neck Core Lifts		
Integrated Core Work in Chair at Wall		

8

THE EMOTIONAL BRAIN AND THE BREATH

We've explored the biochemistry and biomechanics of breath. Now we shift to the third and equally important factor that informs our breath patterns: the impact of our thoughts and feelings on how we breathe. We will explore how our breath impacts our psycho-emotional tone and how our emotions impact our breath. The information in this chapter recaps some of the basic understanding of the nature of the mind laid out by the yogis in Chapters 1 and 2. Here we address it from a Western psychological framework. The practices detailed in this chapter offer an opportunity for you to revisit the relationship between mind and breath, building on the svādhyāya you've cultivated since the beginning of this journey.

Our Brain on Stress

It's sometimes hard to accept the fact that much or even most of the time we are not as happy as it feels like we "should" be. The US Constitution even states that the pursuit of happiness is an unalienable right. Yet, according to neuroscience, in light of humans' development it makes sense that we are less than perfectly happy much of the time. The brain is ever-vigilant, scanning for potential dangers, lurking predators, or anything else that may compromise our life. It does its job regardless of our current desires for happiness. From an evolutionary standpoint, this adaptation served us well in a world where hypervigilance could make the difference between being eaten by predators or survival. Yet hypervigilance tends to create chaos and confusion for many of us living in modern society. Now the predators are often virtual (i.e. fed by the internet). We learn about terrifying events over which we have no direct cause and effect. The news gets amplified by the turnings of our own mind (the vṛttis). As sophisticated as the brain is, it may not discern the difference between an actual event that is happening to us presently and the imagined experience that we've either rehashed from the past or are musing about as a possibility in the future. The internal response from our body to "manufactured" stressors replicates the same response as it would to the experience itself. Our nervous system reacts with a cascade of physiological changes, pushing us into a fear or avoidance reaction. This explains how we can find ourselves in a state of panic even when we are not currently experiencing imminent danger.

The level of stress resilience we exhibit when confronted with adversity has much to do with how well practiced we are at working with the "higher mind" (sometimes described as "executive function"), with awareness, and modulating our thoughts and emotions. Many of us were introduced to the concept of emotional regulation rather late in life. As adults we may find ourselves struggling as we attempt to resolve long-standing fears or tendencies to lash out or shut down entirely when life becomes difficult. Yoga practices can help us to move from a fearful, avoidant-driven reaction and become more stress-resilient by helping us cultivate tools to self-regulate our nervous system. Of all the mechanisms yoga offers in this vein, prāṇāyāma is among the most useful and reliably transformative.

Understanding How We're Wired

The amygdala, a small almond-shaped structure in the limbic brain, plays an integral role in emotional regulation. The amygdala acts as a smoke detector for our fear system. It keeps us safe by kicking us into an immediate reflexive, often defensive, reaction to stimuli that the brain perceives as threatening. This more innate, perhaps less evolved reaction has been described as our "low-road" response, or the response that's quick and easy.[1] If we've spent our lives traversing the low road, we will be expert at imprinting our limbic brain to react negatively to stress. In other words, we'll have carved a deep groove or saṃskāra for interpreting our daily interactions as potential threats. If we regularly freak out when encountering a new situation or person, we will become proficient at avoiding the unfamiliar. Not only does this limit our exposure to new experiences, but it insidiously reinforces that the world is a scary place. The avoidant reaction builds on itself and keeps our sympathetic nervous system (SNS) revved up in fight, flight, or freeze. This is the state the yogis would describe as duḥkha, where we feel powerless and stuck in a rut of our own making.

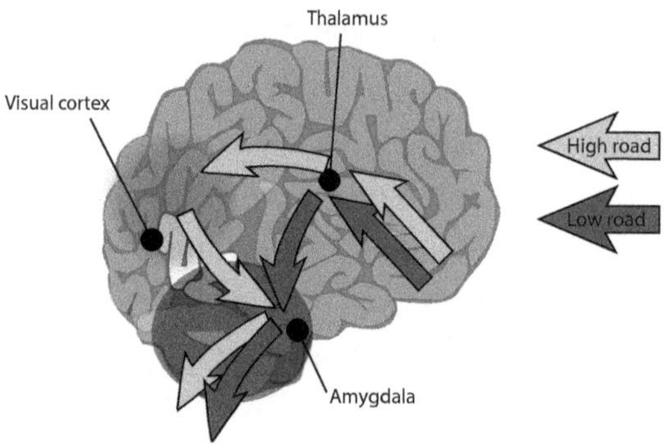

Figure 8.1 High Road/Low Road

In contrast, the prefrontal cortex activates the high road, the path of choice or approach. The prefrontal cortex (PFC) sits at the front of the brain and is largely responsible for directing our cognitive behavior and rational discernment. When our PFC is guiding us, we can think through our fears and respond to stimuli with curiosity, creativity, and positive feeling. The PFC is linked to the parasympathetic nervous system (PNS), also known as the rest-and-digest or tend-and-befriend mode. The PNS is largely regulated by the vagus nerve—a nerve complex that runs from our gut all the way up through our heart and throat, and links to the ears, mouth, and eyes. It partially enervates the diaphragm and is directly affected by the breath. When we coo and rock a distraught baby, softly smiling and gazing into their eyes, we are using our vagal and parasympathetic systems to regulate theirs. Mother–infant bonding is all about wiring up the vagus. It demonstrates the primal means we have to take us out of low-road reactivity into high-road responsiveness and positive social engagement. This level of vagal response releases tension and shifts us into readiness to move forward—in other words, approach.[2]

Body-based practices like yoga are effective ways of activating the calming vagal response. They can be used to transform us from low-road reactors into high-road, approach responders. This is because neural integration happens *top down* (brain to body) and *bottom up* (body to brain). *Neural integration* is a term used for the way we regulate attention, mood, thought, and behavior in response to stimuli.[3] While we are constantly receiving information from the outside via the senses (including the mind), our body is also feeding information back to the brain in the form of muscle tension, gut contraction, heart flutters, and breath patterning. These physical cues are then interpreted by the mind, which fills in the narrative. The mind references times past when the internal, felt sense was similar. The newly constructed story reinforces physiological messages received from the body, thus validating the experience as a whole. If we change our mood, posture, or breath patterns, we can actually alter the entire dialogue between the mind and body. Much like the rocking of a baby, we can wire up our own vagus by moving rhythmically with a calm, parasympathetic-style breathing pattern, perhaps cooing a mantra like "om shanti" to ourselves. Through this kind of process, the body convinces the mind that it is safe, and emotional equilibrium is restored.

As discussed in previous chapters, chronic stress alters our chemistry, affecting heart rate, breath rate, and musculoskeletal tension. Long-standing emotional stress can easily shift us into sympathetic overdrive whereby we essentially forget how to relax and rest. In this state of hyperarousal, we can easily become chronic chest-breathers and low-level hyperventilators. The more emotionally unbalanced we feel, the more we clench our teeth and tighten our chest, and the harder we breathe. The harder it is to breathe, the more stressed we feel. These signals combine to tell the brain that the current state of affairs is indeed overwhelming. In turn, our body locks down defensively, which drives us to gasp for relief. This cyclical pattern makes us more vulnerable to emotional reactivity and less able to make rational, high-road decisions.

The breath offers us a direct means to interrupt this cycle by asserting manual control over the ANS. When we breathe as if everything is okay, the heart rate settles, the muscles relax, and the mind gets the message to change the narrative it has been spinning. In this way, the breath gives us agency to apply the vagal brake[4] and literally change our mental construct and mood. Functional breathing can effectively modulate reactivity while establishing good neural integration. Up until now, the most common way yoga teachers have supported access to the parasympathetic nervous system has been the use of extended exhales. Each time we exhale, heart rate lowers and we pump the PNS. It follows logically, then, that if we wish to self-soothe, we simply extend the exhalation breath for several breath cycles.

Similar to belly breathing, this technique can be useful as an immediate means to calm one who is in a state of panic, acute pain, or anxiety. If relied upon as the sole breath regulation device, it can exacerbate pre-existing physiological imbalance. This is especially true for those already prone to anxiety or asthma, or with a habit of over-breathing. Extended exhales will drop CO_2 levels further and potentially result in feeling less stress resilient and more easily triggered over time. Alternatives offered in this chapter include humming, silent mantra, and the use of short breath holds.

A variety of tools are needed in order to be successful when addressing the psycho-emotional aspect of breath retraining. The most critical aspect for consideration is the nature of the mind of the particular student or client. A breathing technique that is beneficial for one person may be triggering for another. Combining prāṇāyāma with interoceptive and proprioceptive reflections (svādhyāya), as demonstrated throughout this SBJ process, facilitates the construction of a robust neural integration network, and ultimately strengthens the vagal brake.

PRACTICE 8.1: SENSORY SVĀDHYĀYA PRACTICE

In the Katha Upanishad, the analogy of a horse and chariot conveys the relationship between the senses, the emotional mind, and the higher mind of discernment. The horse represents the senses; the reins, the mind pulled by emotions; and the charioteer represents the conscious Self. The question is: Who has control of the reins—the senses or the Self? This teaching represents how we can be pulled by the force of the senses and directed to follow their "scent." The svādhyāya practice articulated below is intended to help you develop more vidya (knowledge), more interoceptive awareness of how the senses and the breath interrelate and "pull" you into an emotionally reactive state. With yoga we are always seeking to develop the conscious Self.

Choose one of the five senses to focus on for a period of time, perhaps over the course of several days or a week. Attend to your response to this sense through your daily activities. If you choose a sound, for instance, observe all sounds: from the birds chirping in the tree, to the crash of the garbage truck. Relay this information through the lens of the breath. In other words, what happens to your breath when you listen and feel the impact of this sound on your nervous system? Reflect on these interoceptive questions and add any others that you think of at the bottom of the list:

- Does your breath speed up or slow down?
- Does it become shallower and/or chest-driven?
- Does it become deeper, more abdominally-diaphragmatically driven?
- Does it stop altogether?
- How does this information help you to understand how this sense affects your emotions and state of mind?
- Are there particular vṛttis (thoughts/feelings/sensations) that accompany your approach-or-avoid response to this sound (or sight, taste, touch, smell)?
- Can you move beyond the reflex of like/don't like and become curious as to how this sensory event impacts you?
- If you change your breathing does it change your relationship to the sensory event?

____

____

Use the space below to track your observations of the relationship between your senses and your breath. Once you have completed this for one sense, follow through with each of the others. Complete the process by using the mind (informational input) as the sixth sense. The intention at this stage is not to change your reaction but rather to notice—witness—it; that is to say, observe it unfolding within you.

Sense to be Observed: ____________________

Day 1 Date __________ Observations

____

____

Day 2 Date __________ Observations

____

____

Day 3 Date __________ Observations

____

____

Day 4 Date __________ Observations

____

____

Day 5 Date __________ Observations

____

____

Day 6 Date __________ Observations

____

____

Day 7 Date __________ Observations

____

____

Sense to be Observed: ____________________

Day 1 Date __________ Observations

____

____

Day 2 Date __________ Observations

____

____

Day 3 Date __________ Observations

____

____

Day 4 Date __________ Observations

____

____

Day 5 Date __________ Observations

____

____

Day 6 Date __________ Observations

____

____

Day 7 Date __________ Observations

____

____

Sense to be Observed: ____

Day 1 Date ____________ Observations

____

____

Day 2 Date ____________ Observations

____

____

Day 3 Date ____________ Observations

____

____

Day 4 Date ____________ Observations

____

____

Day 5 Date ____________ Observations

____

____

Day 6 Date ____________ Observations

____

____

Day 7 Date ____________ Observations

____

____

Sense to be Observed: ____________________

Day 1 Date ________ Observations

____

____

Day 2 Date ________ Observations

____

____

Day 3 Date ________ Observations

____

____

Day 4 Date ________ Observations

____

____

Day 5 Date ________ Observations

____

____

Day 6 Date ________ Observations

____

____

Day 7 Date ________ Observations

____

____

Sense to be Observed: ______________________________

Day 1 Date __________ Observations

____

____

Day 2 Date __________ Observations

____

____

Day 3 Date __________ Observations

____

____

Day 4 Date __________ Observations

____

____

Day 5 Date __________ Observations

____

____

Day 6 Date __________ Observations

____

____

Day 7 Date __________ Observations

____

____

Sense to be Observed: ____________________

Day 1 Date __________ Observations

____

____

Day 2 Date __________ Observations

____

____

Day 3 Date __________ Observations

____

____

Day 4 Date __________ Observations

____

____

Day 5 Date __________ Observations

____

____

Day 6 Date __________ Observations

____

____

Day 7 Date __________ Observations

____

____

When you have completed the process outlined above, use the space provided below to summarize your overall experience of this practice. What have you learned overall about your relationship with your sensory system?

At this point, go back through your Energy Bank Account (EBA) reflections from Chapter 2. Re-evaluate your experience of the panchavāyus (five winds). Explicitly connect the senses and the mind to your EBA observations and reflect on the following questions. Use the space provided below for your responses.

- What have you learned about how the senses govern your EBA?

- How much of your energy is consumed by your senses? Do all of the senses equally consume energy or are you driven by some more than others?

- How can this svādhyāya process on the senses help you make different lifestyle and behavioral choices to bring your EBA more in balance?

PRACTICE 8.2: WIRING UP THE VAGUS SERIES—BREATH PRACTICES TO TRANSFORM THE MIND

The following breathing practices offer effective alternatives to the use of extended exhalation as a means to calm the nervous system. The first few come from the Vedic tradition. The use of short breath holds (SBH) is from the Buteyko method. I have found each of these to be useful in varying contexts and, like anything, no single modality will work for everyone. Experiment, explore, and track your experience using the Breath Practice Chart provided below.

(A) Brahmari—the Bee Breath or Humming

Brahmari, or Bee Breath, refers to the vibrational sound that is created when we hum. Close your lips, place your tongue on the roof of your mouth, and hum at any pitch or vibration that feels comfortable. Humming can be loud or soft, high or low. Experiment and notice how you feel and how you breathe when you hum. The use of sound and mantra have long been recognized as soothing to the nervous system. That said, brahmari is the only type of sound-making that also ensures nasal breathing, as your mouth must be closed in order to hum.

I have recommended brahmari for chronic mouth breathers, encouraging them to sprinkle it in throughout their day regardless of where they are. It is extremely beneficial as a way of increasing consciousness of the breath while keeping their lips together. Brahmari also provides an opportunity to practice proper tongue placement at the upper palate. It can easily be woven into āsana practice, particularly with dynamic movement. The hum can initiate any movement done on an exhale, such as lowering the arms or forward-bending.

Here are some ideas for how to "play" with brahmari, linking it to the concepts communicated in this and previous chapters:

- Play with the coordination of your core muscles and brahmari: Does humming activate the engagement of your abdominals and diaphragm any differently?
- Play with pitch: Can you feel a different resonance in your annamaya (physical body) with higher or lower pitches?
- How does your tongue push against your palate when you hum? Lightly? Forcefully? Equally left and right?
- Play with volume: How is it different to hum loudly, or softly, or softer still?
- Play with brahmari as an "emergency intervention" to interrupt the vṛttis (thoughts/feelings/sensations) when you find yourself sliding down the low road: What do you notice? Is it an effective intervention for you?
- How does brahmari affect your attention and your prāṇa? Do you feel more rajasic (agitated), tamasic (lethargic), or sattvic (light/balanced) during and after practice?

Note: Your experience after the practice may differ in energy from the feeling you experience during practice.

If you have a headache, please refrain from this practice.

(B) Silent Mantra

"Mantra" means to transcend or protect us from our ordinary mind. The use of a phrase or single word as a mantra is a beautiful practice for transforming the vṛttis. It replaces our negative thoughts with something sattvic and links us to that. Whether we are feeling mentally depressed and need to invoke "Light" (om jyoti namaha), or we are feeling anxious and need to connect the grounding force of the earth (om prithivī namaha), mantra has the power to shift our mind out of its neurotic loops and return us to our center.

The Vedic teaching on mantra is vast and this brief descriptor is not in any way intended to illuminate that body of work. What is offered here is more of a simple way to link *bhāvana* (meaning or intention) with the breath, to offer you reprieve from mental agitation or duḥkha. There are four phases to the breath: inhale; retention; exhale; suspension. Each one activates the panchavāyus in its own way. Mantra can be utilized to emphasize just one side of the breath, as in chanting out loud in order to effectively slow down and extend the exhale. Silent mantra can be activated on any or all phases of the breath depending on the desired effect.

Inhalation and hold after inhale (retention) are considered more energizing. Activating mantra with these two breath phases is useful if the mind is sluggish and tamasic or stuck on a negative loop, as can happen with depression. Exhale and hold after exhale (suspension) has more of a quieting effect. Combining mantra with them can help to still the "pinball" mind associated with anxiety. In addition, suspension positively affects CO_2 levels and oxygenation as discussed in previous chapters. When held for short periods, suspension has a parasympathetic effect on the nervous system. When held longer, it produces a mixed effect on the ANS. This will be explained more fully in Chapter 10 as we explore kumbhāka, or longer breath holds.

Note: The term *holding the breath* can itself be triggering for some people. Suspending the breath has a different feel to it. Some people may prefer other options, like "pausing" or "resting between breaths."

Lynn Gorton, a Buteyko colleague and pulmonary rehabilitation specialist, shared the way she uses mantra to help her patients in the hospital clinic. Lynn works with people with severe COPD, many of whom are on oxygen tanks. These people often experience a feeling of panic when attempting breath control practices. Lynn believes strongly in the mind–body–spirit connection and has found that adding the following mantra provides solace to many of her patients, calming fear as it arises. Each word is to be recited silently and timed with the breath.

- Inhale: Peace.
- Retention (hold after inhale): Amen.
- Exhale: Chaos (release the inner turmoil).
- Suspension (hold after exhale): Hallelujah.

Notice that with Lynn's mantra, the shortest side of the breath is the inhale; the longest is suspension. This is in keeping with the desired effect of recalibrating CO_2 levels and avoiding hyperventilation. Lynn's example illustrates that simple one- or two-word mantras can be extremely powerful and need not be in Sanskrit. While om shanti (bless me with peace) is lovely, not everyone is comfortable using a language other than their own. Thich Nhat Han offers many simple mantras of this type in his books on breathing meditations. I often use Light, Love, Joy, and Peace, individually or in combination.

Note: If you are at all concerned that you may be a low-level hyperventilator or over-breather, I would recommend refraining (for a period of time) from chanting out loud, and utilize either brahmari or silent mantra as alternatives. This is particularly important for those engaged in a regular chanting practice.

(C) Halo Breathing (Photo 100)

This practice was introduced to me by a very dear colleague, Matra Majmundar, known as "The Breathing Lady" in the cardio-pulmonary community in which she serves. Matra is a respiratory occupational therapist and yoga therapist. She regularly uses Halo Breathing with her patients, even those who are on oxygen, and finds they respond very positively to it. In particular, they cite its immediate, calming effect on their breathing. Halo breathing is created through a circular rotation of the head. The movement creates an almost trancelike feeling that people describe as meditative and soothing. It has become my personal favorite way to practice Subtle Breathing, as it seems to effortlessly reduce both breath rate and volume. Halo breathing is particularly helpful if you have attempted to reduce your breath and found the process stressful.

1. Prepare yourself as you would for seated Subtle or Core Breathing.
2. Visualize a small "halo" a few inches above your crown center.
3. Begin to roll your head gently in a circle to trace the halo.
4. Your head will oscillate slightly at your occiput.
5. Every 5–6 rotations, reverse direction (clockwise/counterclockwise).
6. Notice that one direction of rotation may feel more comfortable to you initially.
7. Observe what happens naturally to your breathing.
8. Let the breath minimize until you feel a slight sense of air hunger. Continue rotating.
9. Sustain the rotation, changing directions periodically, for 4–5 minutes.
10. Relax your breath and observe the effect.

Repeat 2–3 more rounds of Halo Breathing with breath reduction and slight air hunger for 4–5 minutes.

Notice the felt sense of working with the Halo. How is it different? How does your breathing change in rate or volume?

____

____

What's your feeling at the end of the practice?

____

____

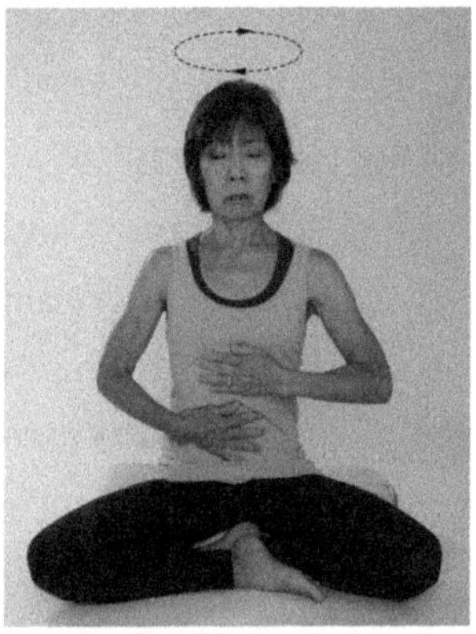

Photo 100

Note: If you find yourself getting dizzy while doing the Halo Breathing, I suggest you try with your eyes open. If that doesn't help, discontinue this practice.

(D) Short Breath Holds (SBH) with Movement (Photos 101 and 102)

This practice is an extremely useful technique for multiple conditions. I use it regularly for students with a low Comfortable Pause (CP) (below 15), or those with anxiety who are just getting started with breath work. Sometimes I use it personally if I've been lecturing a lot and am aware that my CP is low, before I go into my regular prāṇāyāma practice. One of the beautiful things about the SBH practice is that it tends to be less anxiety-producing than longer breath holds. Combined with movement, it can actually be doubly useful in application of the vagal brake. SBH practice can be done multiple times a day as a formal practice, or as an emergency stop-gap measure to quell feelings of anxiety, stress, or panic that arise circumstantially.

1. Take your CP (see Chapter 3).
2. Sit or stand comfortably.
3. Gently inhale and exhale through your nose.
4. Pinch your nose and hold for no more than half of your CP (e.g. if CP was 10 seconds, start your first SBH at 5). If you don't know your CP, start with a hold of 5 seconds.

5. While holding your breath, sway from side to side.
6. Between rounds, pause the movement and take 1–2 small, silent resting breaths through your nose.
7. With the next round of SBH, increase the hold by 1–2 seconds as able, without pushing yourself into a gasp with the subsequent inhalation.
8. Continue to build the holds slowly and progressively.
9. Play with the movement:
   - If sitting, you can undulate in figure 8s or "chair-dance."
   - If standing, you can march, jog in place, or dance free-form.
10. Remember that as you move you are creating more CO_2, which will intensify the experience.
11. Do 6–8 repetitions of SBH.
12. Relax your breath and observe the effect.

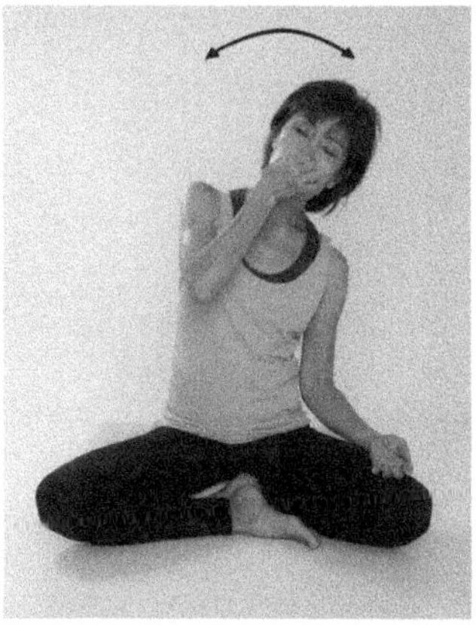

Photo 101

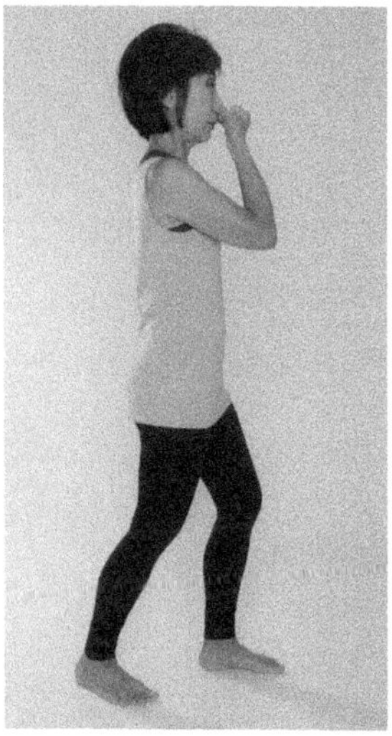

Photo 102

Note: As you gradually build your breath holds, ensure that you are always able to take a relaxed breath through your nose on the inhalation that follows, without gasping. Also, be sure to take enough resting breaths in between reps to allow your breath to settle. If you jump into the next rep too soon, your breath-hold time will likely be lower. If this happens, just relax your breath, let it completely normalize, and then begin again.

Contraindications: If you are pregnant, have uncontrolled high blood pressure, have had a heart attack or stroke in the last three months, have an aneurysm of the aorta or in your brain, kidney disease, arrhythmia, or tachycardia, or have very low lung function on a baseline spirometry test, *please refrain from this practice.*

(E) Combination Practice

1. Try interspersing a round of SBHs in between rounds of seated Subtle or Core Breathing.
2. Do 4 minutes of Subtle or Core Breathing.
3. A round of SBH (6–8 repetitions).
4. Another 4 minutes of Subtle or Core Breathing.
5. Another round of SBH (start where you left off at the last round and build for another 6–8 cycles).
6. Finish with a round of Subtle or Core Breathing.
7. Observe and feel, letting the breath relax.
8. Wait a few minutes until your breathing normalizes.
9. Take your CP and notice how it has been affected by the practice.

Once you have a sense of the practices detailed above, mix and match them with the practices suggested in previous chapters. For example, add Brahmari or Silent Mantra to the core practices described in Chapter 7, or interweave the diaphragmatic practices in Chapter 6 with SBH. What do you notice? Track your combined observations using the chart below.

Charting Breath Practices to Transform the Mind

Write a brief description of your experiences with these practices in the chart below as you explore them over the next month.

Use the space below the chart to describe your overall experience with this process and your svādhyāya on the relationship between the breath and the mind.

Breath Practice Chart

Week 1

Type of Practice	Frequency	Reflections on Practice
Brahmari		
Silent Mantra (Describe mantra)		
Halo Breathing		
Short Breath Holds (SBH) with Movement		
Combination Practice (Describe your process)		

Week 2

Type of Practice	Frequency	Reflections on Practice
Brahmari		
Silent Mantra (Describe mantra)		
Halo Breathing		
Short Breath Holds (SBH) with Movement		
Combination Practice (Describe your process)		

Week 3

Type of Practice	Frequency	Reflections on Practice
Brahmari		
Silent Mantra (Describe mantra)		
Halo Breathing		
Short Breath Holds (SBH) with Movement		
Combination Practice (Describe your process)		

Week 4

Type of Practice	Frequency	Reflections on Practice
Brahmari		
Silent Mantra (Describe mantra)		
Halo Breathing		
Short Breath Holds (SBH) with Movement		
Combination Practice (Describe your process)		

9

THE MIND OF THE SUBTLE BODY

As was established in previous chapters, breath and mind symbiotically chase one another. Prāṇāyāma facilitates the settling of both. In this chapter, we dip further into the relationship between the mind, the breath, and the senses from the hatha yoga tradition. The practices in this section detail various prāṇāyāma techniques from hatha yoga that utilize chakra imagery and *bija* (seed) mantra practices that support bringing the breath and mind into sattvic balance.

The Manomaya Kosha up Close

According to the yoga teachings, there are three primary aspects of the mind, and each plays a unique role in our self-perception: *Manas* is the sensory relay center that takes in information via the senses, which includes the taking in of information through the mind itself; *ahaṃkāra*, or the "I-maker" as it is translated, makes sensory input relevant to the self; *buddhi* discerns what to do with that information, acting in essence as the "decider." The interplay of the senses and their impact on our thoughts, feelings, and subsequent action formulate a guiding principle in yoga. This differs from the Western orientation to mind which tends to view thought and feeling as separate experiences, and rarely examines how often our actions are motivated by our senses. Although buddhi acts in ways reflective of the prefrontal cortex, this wisdom-mind is said to reside in the heart, not in the head. The ancient teachings emphasize that the health of the mind and heart are interdependently woven together.

Classical and hatha yoga both place great importance on the impact of the senses on our psycho-emotional responses. These traditions recognize that strong emotional reactivity to stimuli strengthens the power of the senses to entice us. This keeps us locked in a dualistic dance of desire and aversion. You could think of this as another way of understanding approach and avoid. Practices that refine or reinterpret our relationship to the senses have a neutralizing effect on the mind. Patañjali defines *pratyāhāra*, the fifth of his eight-limbed approach to practice, as the refinement or withdrawal of the senses from external sources. The practice of pratyāhāra helps us to direct our attention away from sensory gratification or repulsion. Prāṇāyāma facilitates the development of pratyāhāra, and is therefore considered essential to this process.

Hatha Yoga and the Chakra Model

Hatha yoga teaches that easeful flow of prāṇa into and around the heart (known as *hṛdaya* in the texts) promotes healthy heart-mind communication. The more distracted the mind is by sensory input, the less prāṇa flows through the hṛdaya. This hampers our ability to attune ourselves to the breath, to quiet the mind, and to achieve the state of meditation. Hatha yoga practices seek to balance the polar energies within us through the engagement of the senses in a more internal, introspective manner. Āsana, prāṇāyāma, mantra, mūdra, and visualization are primary mediums used in the hatha yoga tradition for this purpose. *Prāṇa vidya* (knowledge of prāṇa), *prāṇa shakti* (great prāṇic energy), and *kundalini rising* (the release of the serpent power of wisdom) are different Sanskrit terms used to describe the achievement of prāṇic balance when duality ceases. The goal of hatha yoga is to cultivate this state of unitive consciousness.

The three major energy channels or *nādis* through which prāṇa flows are *iḍā*—left, *piṅgalā*—right, and *suṣumnā*—the central channel (see the box below) There are more than 72,000 nādis flowing through our body. Eventually, they each flow into piṅgalā or iḍā, which are represented as the "sun" and "moon" channels. The major chakra centers form the intersecting points where these two primary nādis coalesce with suṣumnā. Iḍā and piṅgalā have been correlated with the parasympathetic and sympathetic aspects of the nervous system, although studies are not wholly conclusive on this topic. Prāṇāyāma nostril techniques are intended to regulate prāṇa, by channeling the breath through one or both primary nādis, in a process of recalibration.

THE THREE PRIMARY NĀDIS

- **iḍā:** Begins at the left nostril and runs through each of the seven primary chakra centers. It is linked to the myelinated PNS. Qualities: Cooling, quieting, feminine, receptive energies. It is called the chandra or moon channel.
- **piṅgalā:** Begins at the right nostril and runs through each of the seven primary chakra centers. It is linked to the SNS. Qualities: Heating, stimulating, masculine, assertive energies. It is called the sūrya or sun channel.
- **suṣumnā:** Begins at the base of the spine and runs through each of the seven primary chakras. It is centrally located in the spinal column. When the energy of iḍā and piṅgalā are in balance, it is said that we are functioning from suṣumnā. Described as prāṇa shakti, or prāṇa vidya, when the flow of energy is moving through suṣumnā, it is thought that the PNS and SNS are balanced. This produces a sense of alert calm, focused presence, and relaxed clarity.

The Chakra Centers—Then and Now

Modern-day chakra practice and theory are often fraught with misinterpretation. In the original hatha yoga texts, these centers represented areas where toxicity (*ama*) tended to collect, thus obstructing the practitioner's ability to achieve the state of enlightenment, known as *samādhi*. The intent was to drive prāṇa from the periphery into suṣumnā nādi and clear out the ama. Mantra (sound), yantra (gazing techniques), mūdra (hand gestures), and aromatherapy were traditional mediums used to engage the senses, in order to redirect the flow of prāṇa. The elements were also central to these chakra practices, offering a means to directly work with the subtle body and balance the dośas.

Combining prāṇāyāma with these other techniques amplifies the effect of both. Through repetition, the intention to transform the mind and relinquish attachment to the senses is reinforced. The chakra model provides a way of integrating the nervous, endocrine, and sensory systems with the mind and the elements to achieve psychophysiological balance, and ultimately spiritual transcendence. The combination of prāṇāyāma nostril techniques with the bhāvana (intention) of connecting to the chakras can be a very powerful means to direct prāṇa and attention. Below is a summation of the seven primary chakras, following the most familiar model utilized in the West. The chakra centers are commonly correlated with specific colors as specified below. This is a modern Western construct, not reflective of the original yogic texts (see Figure 9.1).

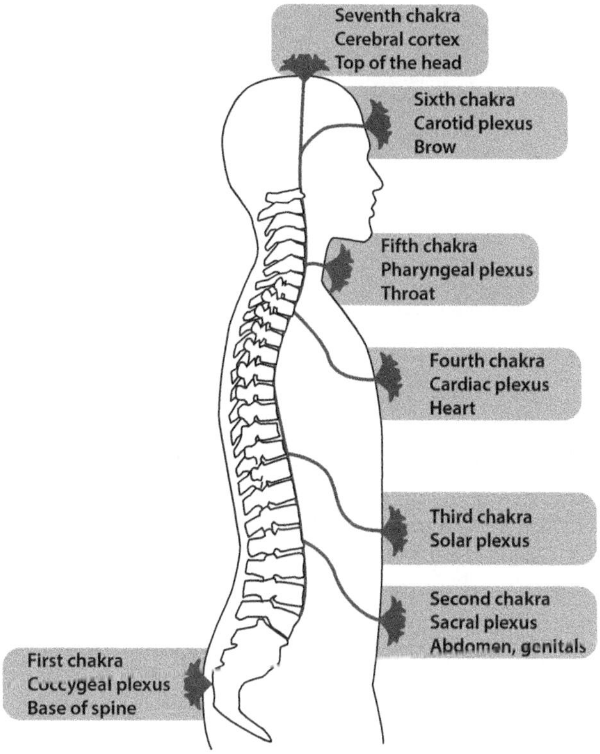

Figure 9.1 Chakras and Nerve Plexuses

Mūladhāra

- First chakra: Root center
- Governs: security, basic survival, and trust
- Endocrine system: sex hormones and adrenals
- Nerve plexus: coccygeal
- Vāyu: apāna (eliminatory)
- Sense: smell

- Element: earth
- Bija mantra: lam
- Designated color: red/black

Svādhiṣṭhāna

- Second chakra: Procreative center
- Governs: sexuality, creativity, boundaries, duality as in pleasure and pain
- Endocrine system: reproductive hormones, adrenals, serotonin
- Nerve plexus: sacral
- Vāyu: vyāna (assimilation)
- Sense: taste
- Element: water
- Bija mantra: vam
- Designated color: orange

Maṇipūra

- Third chakra: Abode of the Self
- Governs: self-empowerment and differentiation
- Endocrine system: insulin, dopamine, serotonin
- Nerve plexus: celiac/enteric
- Vāyu: samāna (digestion)
- Sense: sight
- Element: fire
- Bija mantra: ram
- Designated color: yellow

Anahata

- Fourth chakra: Center of hṛdaya
- Governs: higher emotions such as courage, compassion, empathy

- Endocrine system: thymus gland
- Nerve plexus: brachial
- Vāyu: prāṇa (ingestion)
- Sense: touch
- Element: air
- Bija mantra: yam
- Designated color: green/pink

Viśhuddhi

- Fifth chakra: Center of communication
- Governs: self-expression, truth, and communication (including listening)
- Endocrine system: thyroid
- Nerve plexus: cervical
- Vāyu: udāna
- Sense: hearing
- Element: space
- Bija mantra: ham
- Designated color: turquoise

Ajña

- Sixth chakra: Center of svādhyāya
- Governs: balance between intellect and intuition; development of higher levels of consciousness, meditative focus and introspection
- Endocrine system: pituitary gland
- Bija mantra: ām (ahm)
- Designated color: indigo/violet

Sahāsrara

- Seventh chakra: Spiritual center
- Governs: connection to God or Spirit; center of divine communion

- Endocrine system: pineal gland
- Bija mantra: om
- Designated color: gold/white

PRACTICE 9.1: SVĀDHYĀYA ON THE CHAKRAS

Return to the practices from Chapters 6 and 7. This time, practice them while bringing attention to the specific chakras that are associated with them. Notice how prāṇa is moving through them. For example, with Core Breathing bring particular attention to your first and second chakras. When working with Diaphragmatic Hugs, focus on your third. While doing Scapular Swirls, contemplate your relationship with your fourth chakra. With Paint the Floor, focus on your fifth and perhaps your sixth (especially Paint the Floor with your forehead). Consider these reflective questions as you move and explore:

- How does your prāṇa feel in these areas? Is it rajasic (activated)? Tamasic (lethargic)? Sattvic (balanced)?
- Does bringing attention to your chakra change your movement or your breath?
- How is it to consider your subtle body and flow of prāṇa rather than thinking of just engaging muscles?
- What is the felt sense after your practice?
- Does practicing this way have a different effect on your mind?
- How does practicing with this awareness affect your svādhyāya of your subtle body off the mat?

Utilize the space below to reflect on the felt sense of this exploration of your subtle body, spawned by the questions listed above.

Note: If this type of practice inspires you, try bringing in a little brahmari (humming), or a mantra or mūdra specifically oriented around the chakras (suggestions listed below) and observe the effect.

PRACTICE 9.2: COLORING OUR SENSES

The colors of the rainbow have been associated with the chakra centers. This is a rather "new age" idea that doesn't exactly portray the intention of the yoga scholars, nor does it necessarily resonate as true for each of us as individuals. In the previous chapter, you had the opportunity to play with the senses and notice your relationship to them. Color and our visual sense can greatly impact us. The following practices invite you to focus specifically on color and observe how you relate to color in your environment. Notice what combinations are soothing, and which are more neutral, exciting, or offensive. Do you have a visceral or embodied response to color? If so, where in your body do you experience this? Do all colors impact the same area of your body in the same way?

(A) Colour Play

Use the space below to play with color. Using paints, colored pencils, pastels, or crayons give yourself permission to doodle—not to create a particular design, but rather to observe your response to the colors and combinations of colors on the page. Notice your breath as you play. Write a brief summary of your reflections on this process using the space provided.

(B) Chakra Practice with Color

- Begin to explore bringing color as a visualization aid into your chakra practice. Without a preconceived idea of what specific colors "mean" symbolically, allow yourself to feel where and how your body responds to various tones. For example: Imagine being painted marine blue or fire-engine red. What is your felt experience?

- Attune to the chakra centers specifically and notice if you have a different felt sense/relationship to the centers as you "color" them. For example: Does imagining your third chakra marine blue feel different from painting it fire-engine red? What feels more sattvic to you? What is the prāṇic effect? Go through each of your centers and observe the color pattern that feels in alignment with you. Use the space provided below to reflect on your chakra color experience.

PRACTICE 9.3: CHAKRA BIJA MANTRA PRACTICE

According to the Upanishads, mantra can be a single word or a string of words. Mantra, which literally means to transcend or transform the mind, has been used for many different purposes. It can improve concentration and memory, prepare one for meditation, or facilitate connection to the Divine. In this practice, we are using mantra to activate more awareness of the chakra centers, and the impact of the resonance of sound itself on the breath. The traditional bija or seed mantras for the chakras are as follows, from the bottom up:

Pronunciation note: All of these "a" sounds are pronounced "ah," as in "calm."

- 1st: lam
- 2nd: vam
- 3rd: ram
- 4th: yam
- 5th: ham
- 6th: am
- 7th: om

These can be recited silently or out loud on exhale. Keep the volume of the breath low and controlled via the diaphragm. You can bring these mantras into your āsana and prāṇāyāma practice, focusing on just one at a time or on the full range. Notice how pitch, pace, and volume affect your felt sense of how prāṇa moves within your body.

Reflect on these questions after you have time experimenting with the sounds and vibration in your body.

- How do the vibrations of the sounds resonate inside of you?
- Are some more powerful than others?
- How does this bija chakra focus affect your practice, specifically your mind and your breath?
- What is the overall prāṇic effect (e.g. rajasic, tamasic, sattvic)?
- How has practice impacted your nervous system?
- How effective was this practice for you as a means to quiet both prāṇa and citta?

Use the space provided below to reflect on your experience with the bija mantra practice.

PRACTICE 9.4: MŪDRA AND THE NĀDIS (PHOTOS 103–104)

For centuries mūdras have been used as a way to harness and direct the natural expression of the mind, heart, and spirit. These symbolic gestures made with the hands or other parts of the body activate intention and can be used to amplify the effect of our practice. Chakra practices often incorporate the use of mūdra as a means to connect to the nādis and direct the flow of prāṇa. There is evidence that utilization of mūdras affects the nervous system and alters psychophysiological processes within the body and mind. When working with mūdras, each person must discern through direct experience what is true and useful for him- or herself.

There are many wonderful books that offer illustrations and many details for working with mūdras. My two personal favorites are Joseph and Lilian Le Page's book *Mūdras for Healing and Transformation*, and Indu Arora's *Mūdra: The Sacred Secret*.[1] I would suggest starting your exploration of mūdra by equipping yourself with one of these texts. Choose a specific bhāvana. Use the mūdra within your prāṇāyāma practice and observe the effect. Stay with one mūdra for a period of time (perhaps a few weeks to a month) so you have time to observe the effect. Notice how it impacts your nervous system, your level of reactivity, your breath, and your mind.

Below are a few mūdra suggestions to get you started:

- Choose an elemental mūdra to work with, e.g. Prithivī Mūdra (earth element).
- Choose a vāyu mūdra to work with, e.g. Prān Mūdra, or Apāna Mūdra (Photo 103 Prān Mūdra; Photo 104 Apāna Mūdra).

- Choose a particular mūdra that correlates with a chakra center, e.g. Svādhiṣṭhāna Mūdra.
- Choose a mūdra for balancing the nādis, e.g. Iḍā Mūdra.

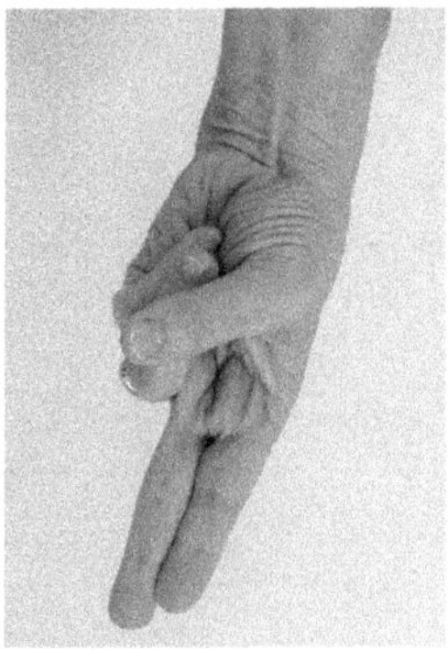

Photo 103

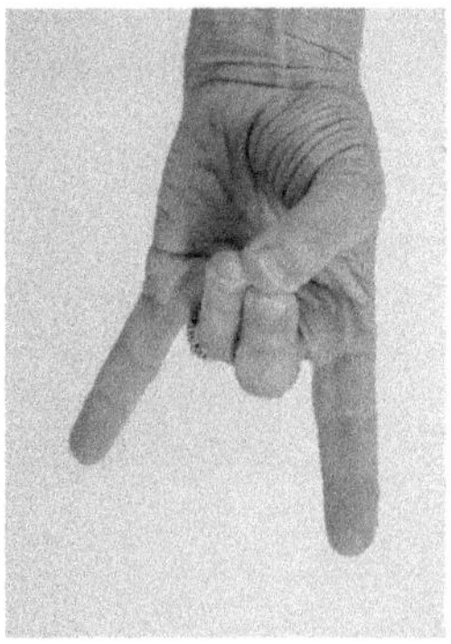

Photo 104

Use the chart provided to describe your experience with mūdra practice over the next month.

Mūdra Chart

Description of Mūdra	Frequency	Reflections on Practice

Description of Mūdra	Frequency	Reflections on Practice

Description of Mūdra	Frequency	Reflections on Practice

Description of Mūdra	Frequency	Reflections on Practice

PRACTICE 9.5: COMBINING MANTRA, MŪDRA, PRĀṆĀYĀMA, AND ĀSANA

This type of approach to practice could be particularly useful for someone who is interested in cultivating the qualities of grounding and stabilization, with an awareness of their first and second chakras.

Combine mantra and mūdra with breath to fortify your intention. For example:

- āsana: seated meditation posture with engagement of the core muscles
- prāṇāyāma: Core Breathing
- mantra: "om prithivī namaha" recited silently on the hold after exhale
- mūdra: Prithivī Mūdra.

Use the chart below to describe your mūdra combination experience. See example provided.

EXAMPLE

Prāṇāyāma and Mudra Combination Chart

Description of Practice	*Frequency*	*Reflections on Practice*
Meditated with Core Breathing and SBH, holding Prithivī Mūdra and chanting silently on breath suspension, "Om prithivī namaha." I also put a picture of Mt. Rainier on my mat—to further invoke the feeling of solidity and groundedness.	*Every day for a week in morning; 10 minutes.*	*Life has been super chaotic this week so I liked the idea of grounding and working with the element of earth. I found it to be very pleasant and focusing. The breath suspension with the mantra makes it easier to hold and I don't feel as anxious doing it. I found by mid-week I was really looking forward to starting my day with this. Seems like even though things are coming at me, it's easier for me to deal with it all. I might continue with this practice for another week.*

Prāṇāyāma and Mudra Combination Chart

Description of Practice	Frequency	Reflections on Practice

Description of Practice	Frequency	Reflections on Practice

Description of Practice	Frequency	Reflections on Practice

Nostril Techniques

As your breath exploration takes you back into the familiar territory of traditional prāṇāyāma practices, it is important to bring the svādhyāya that you have developed through the preceding practices with you. This means to maintain a functional breath, at low volume, moving in the direction of ever more internal attunement. Manipulating the airflow at the nostrils reduces the breath by half, and works deeply with the subtle body, balancing the nādis. These techniques are very useful, *provided that volume and flow rate aren't increased* when the seal is applied. This takes considerable time to master!

Nostril techniques funnel energy through the two primary nādis:

- **piṅgalā:** sūrya/sun, heating, SNS, stimulating
- **iḍā:** chandra/moon, cooling, PNS, calming.

The intention of these prāṇāyāma practices is to bring the polarity of iḍā and piṅgalā into balance. The process can be addressed in one of two ways. The first is to activate the channel that is deficient (tamasic) by working on that side as you inhale, which will be more stimulating. Or, conversely, sedate the channel that's too rajasic by working with it on the exhalation. It is important to observe not just the right-to-left balance but also the apānavayu (below the diaphragm) to prāṇavayu (above the diaphragm) effect, which also impacts the chakras and the ANS.

For example:

- **chandra bhedana** emphasizes iḍā nādi, stimulating the left side with the inhale
- **anuloma ujjayi** emphasizes the calming effect of the exhale, which is done through both nostrils alternately on the exhale. It emphasizes apānavayu, reducing stress and tension.

To discern the discrete differences between these two requires introspective focus and repetition of practice.

Classically, these kinds of prāṇāyāmas were utilized in concert with mantras and mūdras to further regulate prāṇa through the chakra centers. However, I would suggest starting out slow to ensure that the breath doesn't become hard or feel pushed. The process of training yourself to breathe in this highly reduced manner requires svādhyāya and patience. Remember, the use of ujjayi is also intended to be subtle. Limit yourself to a light contraction of the glottis that increases awareness and positive airway resistance, *without creating any outward sound.*

PRACTICE 9.6: HAND MŪDRA FOR NOSTRIL TECHNIQUES (PHOTOS 105 AND 106)

There are many variations from different traditions for this. The way I learned from the Krishnamacharya tradition involves a seal on one side and a valve on the other. This means the hand is touching on both nostrils at all times, ensuring a higher level of regulation. I suggest you try this method, even if you haven't utilized it before. Observe for yourself if it enables you to be a more precise conductor of prāṇa.

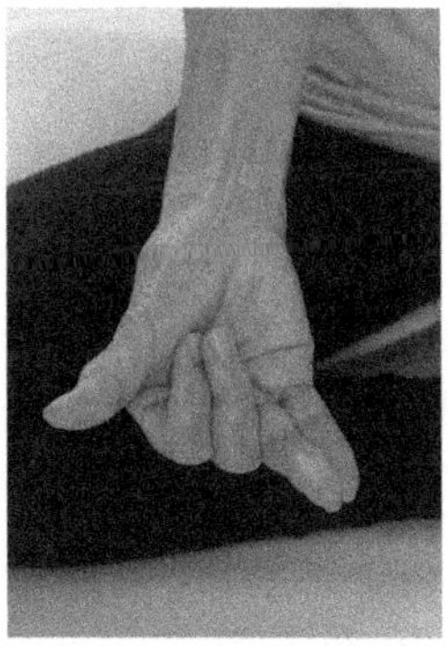

Photo 105

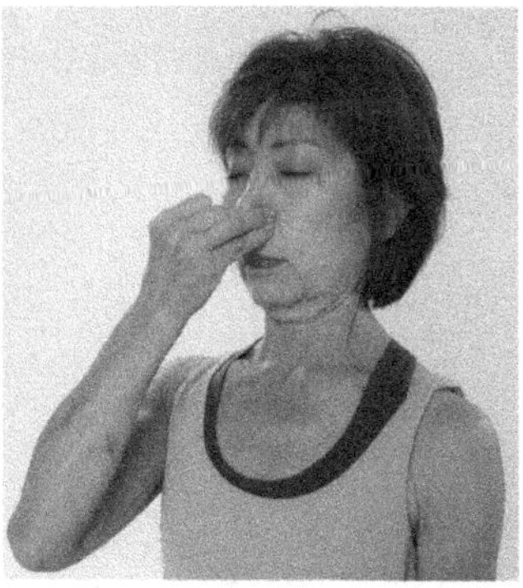

Photo 106

Note: Neck and shoulder tension can make nostril techniques stressful on the annamaya kosha (physical body). If you experience discomfort, try propping with blankets or pillows as shown in Photo 107.

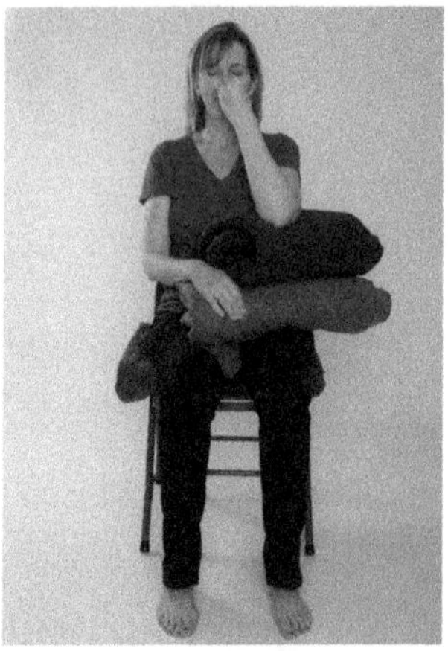

Photo 107

Nādi shodhāna: Alternate nostril breathing. The pattern runs: inhale left; exhale right; inhale right; exhale left. Balancing for both iḍā and piṅgalā with equal emphasis on inhale and exhale. This breath can be beneficial for almost all practitioners.

Viloma ujjayi: Alternate nostril inhale; ujjayi exhale. Viloma ujjayi stimulates the inhalation side of the breath equally on both sides, and as such is an energizing technique. It is beneficial for waking up in the morning, reducing kapha mind, or for a midday pick-me-up. Retention or hold after inhale will amplify the effect of viloma. **Contraindications:** Retention should not be used by anyone who has heart issues or vulnerability to stroke, who is pregnant, or who has high blood pressure.[2]

Anuloma ujjayi: Alternate nostril exhale; ujjayi inhale. Anuloma ujjayi stimulates the exhalation side of the breath equally on both sides and is considered a calming, soothing technique. It is beneficial for quieting the mind when anxious or racy, as it reduces vata (air/ether) and pitta (fire). It is a nice before-bed practice, or done in combination with shītali (the tongue breath), for an added cooling effect. A short suspension after exhale for 4–6 seconds can amplify the quieting effect.

Pratiloma ujjayi: Complex breath. Combines anuloma and viloma ujjayi. The pattern is: inhale ujjayi; exhale left; inhale left; exhale ujjayi; inhale ujjayi; exhale right; inhale right; exhale ujjayi. Four breaths complete one cycle. Pratiloma ujjayi is excellent for ordering the mind and bringing it into focus. It requires great concentration. It is useful for preparing for a mental project or exam, or when you have to juggle many mental "balls." It is not useful for quieting the mind to sleep or rest as it has a highly focusing effect.

Chandra bhedana: Moon breath. Inhale through iḍā (left), exhale through piṅgalā (right), or exhale through iḍā. The focus is specifically on stimulating iḍā nādi. It has an overall calming, cooling effect, and is useful for times of over-stimulation, insomnia, hot flashes and emotional overload; think of it as nourishing and soothing, internalizing attention. Keep the breath flow slow and subtle, maintaining the exhale slightly longer than the inhale (e.g. inhale 4 seconds, exhale 6).

Note: The subject of prāṇāyāma ratios will be addressed in Chapter 10. The above is not a prescribed ratio, but rather a suggestion to keep the exhalation slightly longer than inhalation to maintain a calming, more PNS effect.

Sūrya bhedana: Sun breath. Inhale through piṅgalā (right), exhale through iḍā (left). The focus is specifically on stimulating piṅgalā nādi. It has an overall heating, stimulating effect. This breath may be useful for some kapha conditions, but, for the most part, other practices may be more effective to move prāṇa when it is very sluggish, like going for a brisk walk. Sūrya bhedana can aggravate pitta, which is related to all inflammatory conditions, so it is not one that I recommend on a general basis.

As you explore the nādis and the chakras in these ways, track your experience in the chart provided. Note the effect on your mind, your emotional resilience, and your reactivity to stressors. Observe the prāṇic effects. Experiment with one technique for a long enough period of time that you get a real sense of its effect on your system. Monitor your Comfortable Pause and heart rate for additional information as to how each technique is impacting you. Once you find one or two techniques that seem to have a sattvic effect on your psycho-emotional body, practice them consistently. Observe the therapeutic benefit of these types of practices over the long term.

Use the charts below to track your prāṇāyāma exploration over the next month. The example provides a template for you to follow. Please be sure to use take your Comfortable Pause (CP) and heart rate (HR) both before and after practice for reference. Write your reflection on this type of prāṇāyāma practice in the space provided below the chart.

EXAMPLE

Prāṇāyāma Technique Exploration Chart

Type of Prāṇāyāma Technique	*Time of Day (Typically)*	*CP*	*HR*	*Duration of Practice*	*Number of Days Practiced*	*Intention of Practice—Reason for Choosing*
anuloma ujjaji	*morning*	*20/25*	*72/66*	*20 mins total*	*5x 1st week* *3x 2nd*	*To set my day with more focus and to help calm my anxiety.*

Write your reflections on this prāṇāyāma experience here:

I tend to get anxious about work and rush around in the morning, sometimes feeling like a chicken with my head cut off. I thought AU would be a good way for me have a more relaxed start to my day. I also did six rounds of short breath holds between two 10-minute blocks of AU. The SBH were really helpful last month with my anxiety so I wanted to keep practicing them. I usually do three 10-minute rounds of Core Breathing and SBHs, so I just changed my morning session to AU. I liked it. I found it very soothing and it took more focus than Core or Subtle Breathing. At first I got a little jangled trying to remember which side to close—but that got easier with time. I noticed I felt more clear headed when I got the kids ready for school, and didn't scream at them all week (that's HUGE). I also didn't feel as stressed in traffic on the way to work, which usually sends me off the rails. I'm excited about doing this more. Some days it's just hard to fit it in, especially if I am up late working at night—hard to make myself get up to do my prāṇāyāma in the morning. :(

Prāṇāyāma Technique Exploration Chart

Week 1

Type of Prāṇāyāma Technique	Time of Day (Typically)	CP	HR	Duration of Practice	Number of Days Practiced	Intention of Practice—Reason for Choosing

Write your reflections on this type of prāṇāyāma practice here:

Week 2

Type of Prāṇāyāma Technique	Time of Day (Typically)	CP	HR	Duration of Practice	Number of Days Practiced	Intention of Practice—Reason for Choosing

Write your reflections on this type of prāṇāyāma practice here:

Week 3

Type of Prāṇāyāma Technique	Time of Day (Typically)	CP	HR	Duration of Practice	Number of Days Practiced	Intention of Practice—Reason for Choosing

Write your reflections on this type of prāṇāyāma practice here:

Week 4

Type of Prāṇāyāma Technique	Time of Day (Typically)	CP	HR	Duration of Practice	Number of Days Practiced	Intention of Practice—Reason for Choosing

Write your reflections on this type of prāṇāyāma practice here:

10

PRĀṆĀYĀMA AS KUMBHĀKA

For our culminating chapter and set of practices we now move into the development of breath holds, or kumbhāka. The practices we've worked with thus far were intended to cultivate a level of mental preparedness, as well as establish healthy biomechanical and chemical function in order to successfully explore longer kumbhāka. In multiple yoga texts, prāṇāyāma practice is not differentiated from kumbhāka. The Hatha Yoga Pradipika, for example, mentions eight types of prāṇāyāma; each is named as a type of kumbhāka. Techniques that did not contain breath retention or suspension were not even considered prāṇāyāma. The masters were very clear: The miraculous benefits of prāṇāyāma lay in mastering our volitional power to *not* breathe, nothing more or less than that.

The capacity to suspend the breath for longer periods of time on a regular basis can be developed through progressive reduction of the ventilatory response (the urge to breathe). This is established by consistent lowering of minute volume, proper muscular recruitment, and the refinement of interoceptive awareness. As mentioned earlier, there are four malleable phases of the breath: (1) inhale; (2) retention after inhale; (3) exhale; (4) suspension after exhale. Prāṇāyāma practices orchestrate these in various ratios or patterns to affect the movement of prāṇa, and therefore impact our physiology and our mind in specific ways. Depending on the text or lineage you are referencing, the Sanskrit terms for these phases vary. Attempting to differentiate among the various names and techniques can result in confusion. For clarity, in this text we refer to hold after inhale as retention and hold after exhale as suspension.

Traditionally, the four phases of the breath were measured, creating ratios. The most common means to regulate ratio is numerical counting, as in: inhalation: 4 seconds; retention: 4 seconds; exhalation: 8 seconds; suspension: 4 seconds. Traditionally, mantra was used for this purpose. Shorter or longer mantras would correlate with the phases of the breath. Additionally, mantra weaves in the conceptual element of a specific spiritual or healing intention. As we've explored in previous chapters, mantra can be particularly useful in pacifying the mind and emotions. Retention has certain health precautions associated with it, because holding the breath after inhale can pressurize the thoracic cavity and stress the heart. Suspension is considered safer to practice and is associated with deep states of mental calm. The bandhas were traditionally utilized in prāṇāyāma because they facilitate control of the nervous and circulatory systems, enabling the practitioner to suspend the breath for extended periods of time. The ancient yogis practiced kumbhāka of several minutes at a time, achieving deep states of meditative consciousness (samādhi).[1] In the West and over two millennia after the ancient yogis, Dr. Buteyko formulated his breathing practices to facilitate healing in critically ill patients. Buteyko breathing emphasizes reducing breath volume, and progressively increasing breath suspension for up to 40 seconds.[2]

As we consider the health benefits of breath holding, it is interesting to note that intermittent hypoxia (IH) therapy has been used for the past 30 years with very positive results, ranging from reduction in inflammation and treatment for anxiety and other mental health issues, to increased aerobic fitness and weight loss.[3] IH uses a variety of means to reduce the level of oxygen coming into the body, thus increasing the Bohr effect and giving better oxygenation of the tissues. There are other promising studies looking at the effect of IH on cognitive function, in particular on memory retention. People living at high altitudes, where oxygen levels are lower, have been shown to have fewer heart issues, and lower rates of obesity and diabetes.[4] Athletes who train at high altitude increase speed and endurance times. The culmination of this information substantiates through scientific research many of the health benefits of prāṇāyāma that the yogis have touted for thousands of years.

As encouraging as this is, remember that changing our respiratory chemistry will impact all of our vital functions! Practices that strongly manipulate the blood gases, such as longer kumbhāka, come with a cautionary note. Side-effects can arise if the process is approached too aggressively. There are definite contraindications to extended breath holding: **If you are pregnant, have uncontrolled high blood pressure, have had a heart attack or stroke, have an aneurysm of the aorta or in your brain, arrhythmia or tachycardia, cancer, kidney disease, or very low lung function on a baseline spirometry test, please refrain from these practices.** Additionally, kriyas—cleansing practices such as kapālabhāti (Skull Shining Breath) and bastrika (Bellow's Breath)—have many potential health risks, including exacerbating inflammatory conditions and hyperventilation. These practices are best reserved for specific individuals under the care of a certified yoga therapist (see The Kriyas below).

I strongly suggest, as you embark upon these practices, that you develop a positive samskara of self-monitoring by systematically checking your pulse and CP. This will assist your discernment of the healthy parameters for kumbhāka practice and will go far to keep you in the safe zone. These objective measures provide immediate feedback and can indicate whether prāṇāyāma is taking you towards sattva or pushing you into a rajasic or destabilized state. If your CP after practice is lower than when you began and/or your heart rate is higher, it's an indication that you were pushing your practice beyond your capacity. If you push, you may also experience what is described as a detox effect. With detox, you may experience a temporary aggravation of symptoms, or feel as if you have a cold coming on. You may feel more congested and extra tired for two to three days. If you experience any of these symptoms, I suggest you continue to practice but back off on the intensity of your kumbhāka. Continue to work with a reduced breath and shorter breath holds. Find your equilibrium and then build back up in a more gentle, progressive fashion. If you are working with a teacher or Restore Your Prāṇa mentor, this would be a good thing to discuss with them. The prāṇāyāma charts at the end of this chapter offer you an ongoing tracking tool to support you as you practice.

To experience consistent, beneficial health outcomes through prāṇāyāma, the recommended dose of practice is approximately one hour per day—spread throughout the day, as opposed to doing it in one block. Both the yoga texts and more contemporary methods of breath retraining, such as Buteyko, recommend practicing multiple times a day. This assists the brain's medulla in recalibrating to increase your CO_2 tolerance through consistent reinforcement. Practice can be adapted for your particular lifestyle. For instance, you could choose three 20-minute sessions (morning/midday/evening); four 15-minute sessions with a before-lunch and before-dinner practice in addition to morning and night; or six 10-minute sessions, sprinkled throughout the day. Kumbhāka needs to be practiced on an empty stomach, so always arrange your sessions prior to meals. This orientation provides a kind of flexibility that makes prāṇāyāma accessible for most everyone.

Additionally, kriyas—cleansing practices such as kapālabhāti (Skull Shining Breath) and bastrika (Bellow's Breath)—have many potential health risks, including exacerbating inflammatory conditions and hyperventilation. These practices are best reserved for specific individuals under the care of a certified yoga therapist. The kriyas are more fully addressed below.

The Kriyas: Cleansing Practices

Caution Required! There are a few breath practices that are unique in that they defy the description of extended (*dīrgha*) and subtle (*sūkṣma*). In the texts they are often listed as "kriyas" or "shat-karmas," meaning forceful acts. These are considered cleansing practices, used to reduce phlegm and congestion, and to aid digestion and elimination. These practices require the capacity to engage the muscles of the core with authority. Attempting any of these practices without core awareness and the ability to activate the diaphragm properly with breathing will circumvent any potential benefit to the practice. They are related to both the muscular recruitment needed for bandhas and the ability to sustain kumbhāka. That said, these techniques are not appropriate for most therapeutic students (unless used under the advisement of a trained yoga therapist). While many of them are commonly taught in the yoga community, I encourage you to consider the impact they may have on breathing pattern disorders and common inflammatory conditions before opting to introduce them in group classes.

- **kapālabhāti** (Skull-Shining Breath): Activates the abdominals and diaphragm on the exhale in a forceful, pumping action, "like a blacksmith's bellows." Inhalation is a quick diaphragmatic reflex taken in response. Kapālabhāti, often also referred to as "Breath of Fire," creates a great deal of internal heat, particularly as one becomes more practiced and is able to perform more repetitions in rapid succession. After approximately 50 fast breaths of this type, the breath is held as long as possible. This constitutes one cycle. The instruction is to repeat this cycle until fatigued and then to stop. Traditionally, kapālabhāti is utilized to remove waste products (ama) from the system and to prepare the body for the other prāṇāyāma practices.

- **bastrika** (Bellow's Breath): There are many variations offered of bastrika, depending on the tradition one follows. Within the Hatha Yoga Pradipika there are at least five options given. Similar to kapālabhāti, bastrika is also said to move the breath rapidly, like the blacksmith's bellows. The active movement is taken on the exhale with forceful contraction of the abdominals; however, the inhale requires full expansion of the abdomen. The inhale and exhale are of equal lengths, making it a necessarily bigger breath than kapālabhāti. One of the adaptations of bastrika offered in the Hatha Yoga Pradipika utilizes nostril valving (20 breaths through each nostril) in an alternate fashion. Bastrika moves a larger volume of breath due to the exaggerated inhalation, almost guaranteeing hyperventilation. Each round of rapid breaths is followed by a strong kumbhāka with jālandhara and mūlabandha set in place. Cycles are repeated to the point of fatigue. It is likely these techniques were used by the ancient yogis to off-gas large amounts of CO_2 quickly (short term) in order to increase their kumbhāka and achieve a more acute state of hypoxia. To understand how this works, put it in the context of someone who has a full reservoir of prāṇa, with normal levels of CO_2. In this scenario, their CO_2 tolerance is high. Short-term hyperventilation with a practice such as bastrika will drop CO_2 levels quickly and dramatically. This will allow the practitioner to "marinate" in a kumbhāka for a significantly longer period of time before reaching their threshold. This type of technique is often used among free divers, and in other contemporary breathing practices such as the Wim Hof method.

The kriyas are meant to be used for a specific reason, not simply done as a daily regimen, unless titrated therapeutically. They can be useful for clearing the sinuses (good prep for prāṇāyāma), prompting peristalsis to alleviate constipation, and to activate and strengthen the diaphragm and abdominal core. Unfortunately, they can also exacerbate chronic hyperventilation. It has been postulated that if done correctly, kapālabhāti does not actually cause hyperventilation, as it circulates small amounts of air primarily in the dead space and does not actually disturb blood–gas ratios. The problem is, if one already tends to over-breathe/hyperventilate, the diaphragm is likely to be weak and it will be difficult for the person to create the appropriate pumping action without engaging the accessory muscles and increasing ventilation. Among untrained Westerners, these practices pose a risk of exacerbating pre-existing breathing disorders. This is why I prefer Diaphragmatic and Silent Hugs as described in Chapter 6. These support the conditioning of the diaphragm and visceral motility, without risking the loss of precious amounts of CO_2. Contraindications for kapālabhāti and bastrika are many: high blood pressure, heart disease, brain tumors, stroke, vertigo, stomach or intestinal ulcers, GERD, gastritis, glaucoma, diarrhea, systemic inflammation, and hyperventilation.

PRACTICE 10.1: DEVELOPING SUSPENSION

I like to think of the process of interweaving the Subtle Breathing practices with suspension as a kind of Oreo cookie, with suspension as the creamy middle. Below you'll see scripted options for a 10-, 15-, and 20-minute breathing practice, using this layering concept. Subtle Breathing can be substituted with Core Breathing or Halo Breathing, or any of the nostril techniques you prefer from Chapter 9. Whichever means of working with the Subtle Breath you choose, work to sustain a feeling of slight air-hunger for the duration of the practice. Short breath holds can be interchanged with extended breath holds as is your preference.

The 10-Minute Practice

1. Begin by taking your CP and heart rate (HR).
2. Do 3–4 minutes of seated Subtle Breathing
3. Do 6–8 rounds of short breath holds, building to 20 seconds.
4. Rest for approximately 30 seconds, or until your breath settles.
5. Repeat another 3–4-minute round of seated Subtle Breathing.
6. Rest for 1 minute and let your breath settle.
7. Take your CP and HR. Chart your experience.

The 15-Minute Practice

1. Begin by taking your CP and heart rate (HR).
2. Do 3–4 minutes of seated Subtle Breathing (Core or Halo or Nostril Breathing may also be used).
3. Do 6–8 rounds of short breath holds, building to 20 seconds.
4. Rest for approximately 30 seconds, or until your breath settles.
5. Repeat another 3–4-minute round of seated Subtle Breathing.
6. Take an extended breath hold: Inhale, exhale, pinch your nose, and hold for 5 seconds beyond your CP.
7. Rest for approximately 30 seconds, or until your breath settles.
8. Repeat a third round of Subtle Breathing for 3–4 minutes.
9. Rest for 1 minute and let your breath settle.
10. Take your CP and HR. Chart your experience.

The 20–30-Minute Practice

1. Begin by taking your CP and heart rate (HR).
2. Do 4–5 minutes of seated Subtle Breathing (Core or Halo or Nostril Breathing may also be used).
3. Do 6–8 rounds of short breath holds, building to 20 seconds.
4. Rest for approximately 30 seconds, or until your breath settles.
5. Repeat another 4–5-minute round of seated Subtle Breathing.

6. Take an extended breath hold: Inhale, exhale, pinch your nose, and hold for 5 seconds beyond your CP.
7. Rest for approximately 30 seconds, or until your breath settles.
8. Repeat a third round of Subtle Breathing for 4–5 minutes.
9. Take another extended breath hold. If possible, hold 10 seconds beyond your CP.
10. Rest for approximately 30 seconds, or until your breath settles.
11. Repeat a fourth round of seated Subtle Breathing for 4–5 seconds.
12. Rest for 1–2 minutes and let your breath settle completely.
13. Take your CP and HR. Chart your experience.

Note: When your breath-hold time consistently averages 20 seconds or more, you can replace the SBHs with extended breath holds. Once you are comfortable with the extended kumbhāka, you can work with maximum holds, which are sustained kumbhāka for your maximum capacity, while maintaining nose breathing following the breath suspension. If you gasp or have difficulty settling the breath within 3–4 breaths after your maximum kumbhāka, you held too long and need to modulate with subsequent holds.

If you find "clocking" your suspension via a stopwatch distracting, agitating, or stressful, I suggest finding a soothing mantra that you can repeat that approximates your CP. This will help to keep your attention interiorized and your mind calm. Notice the impact of these more intense practices on your digestion, sleep, appetite, energy levels, mental clarity, and emotional regulation. Always consider the whole panchamaya (five dimensions) in your note-taking, contemplating your prāṇic reservoir, your Energy Bank Account, and the holistic effect of altering your breath in this way.

PRACTICE 10.2: SUSPENSION WITH MOVEMENT SERIES—BREATHE LESS, MOVE MORE!

Practicing suspension during practice is a very productive way to raise your CP. It simulates the action of high-altitude training, or IH therapy, in the sense that you are both raising CO_2 levels through movement and creating a hypoxic effect. I recommend trying these in small doses while walking on a flat surface within your house or around your property. Once you feel the effects and are confident that it is useful for you, you can take it into your regular exercise regime and āsana practice to add a little more challenge to your workout. You may like to use a pulse oximeter to check your oxygen saturation (SpO_2) while you practice. Try to drop your oxygen saturation to below 90 and into the high 80s. Your legs may feel a little rubbery in this process, but you will recover quickly as soon as you breathe normally.

Note: These types of practice are inappropriate for those who have any of the aforementioned contraindications for breath holding.

(A) Walking Practice (Photo 108)

1. Begin with 4–5 minutes of seated Subtle Breathing (Core, Halo, or Nostril Breathing may also be used).
2. Begin to walk, breathing lightly through your nose for 5 minutes.
3. Continue walking and take a short breath hold (SBH), starting with 10 seconds.
4. Always seal both nostrils with your fingers during breath holds.
5. Release the seal, continue walking, and breathe lightly through your nose.
6. Wait until your breath settles before taking the next round.
7. Continue to walk, and when ready take another SBH, holding for 12 seconds.
8. Between rounds of SBH, keep walking at a slow pace, waiting until your breath settles before your next breath hold.
9. Do 6–8 rounds of SBH in this way, building gradually to your comfortable point of challenge.
10. Continue to walk for a while after your last SBH, breathing naturally.
11. After practice, sit and observe your breath for 5 minutes. Notice the effect of your practice.

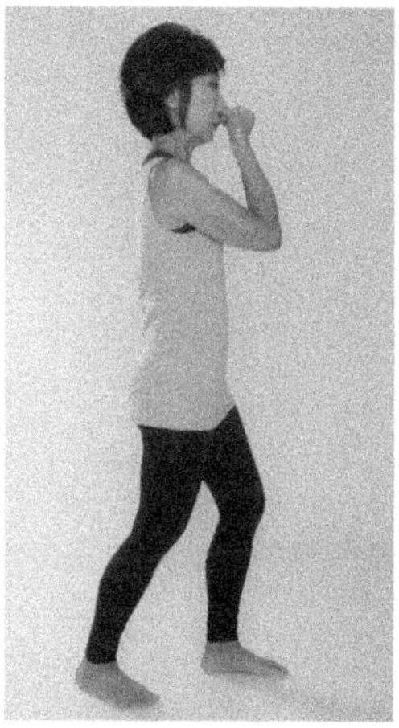

Photo 108

Note: If at any point you feel like you need to rest, please do! Stop walking. Pause. Let your breath settle. It is always better to stop and rest, rather than to push yourself into a large gasp or into a state of agitation. Think of this as walking meditation. You can use a mantra as you walk—after all, it's about being present and observing the breath, not about "getting somewhere."

If you like this process, you can experiment with either of the variations below.

(B) Single Nostril Breathing with Walking

- Close one nostril and continue to walk for 5 minutes, maintaining a subtle volume.
- Take a few relaxed breaths, letting your system settle.
- Change nostrils and walk for another 5 minutes.

(C) Extended Breath Holds with Walking

This practice is best done after you have warmed up with some of the above variations and explored extended breath holds in the seated practice. With this technique, known in the Buteyko Method as "Steps,"[5] you only walk while holding the breath. After each breath hold you pause in stillness. Allow the breath to settle completely between cycles.

1. Warm your body with a brisk 10-minute walk or similar activity.
2. Stand still and settle the breath.
3. Inhale/exhale, seal both nostrils and walk, counting your steps. Start with 10–15 steps.
4. Stop moving and release the seal on your nose. Breathe in through your nose.
5. Let your breath settle.
6. Do another round, holding again for the same number of steps or building by 1–2 steps.
7. Always stop, rest, and settle your breath between rounds. Continue for 6–8 cycles, building gradually and finding your comfortable maximum point of challenge, e.g. 20, 25 steps, etc.

As time allows, complete the moving practice with a seated prāṇāyāma practice of your choosing. Allow 5–10 minutes after this for the breath to completely settle before taking your CP and HR again.

Note: These practices quickly elevate CO_2 levels, which can have a laxative effect on the intestines. This is great news for those with sluggish digestion; however, if you have inflammatory bowel conditions or habitually tend towards diarrhea, I suggest you use these practices judicially, and decide if they are appropriate for you. Once you have a sense of how the regulation of the breath and breath holds work for you with movement, you can institute them in your āsana practice or other exercise regimes.

Use the chart provided below to track your kumbhāka practice. Please be sure to use take your Comfortable Pause (CP) and heart rate (HR) both before and after practice for reference.

Kumbhāka Tracking Chart

Type of Prāṇāyāma Technique	CP before/ after	HR before/ after	Extended or Maximum Kumbhāka	Duration of Practice	Number of Days Practiced	Variations on Practice (e.g. Use of Moving Practices in Combination with Nostril Techniques)
Write your reflection on this type of prāṇāyāma practice here:						
Write your reflection on this type of prāṇāyāma practice here:						

Type of Prāṇāyāma Technique	CP before/ after	HR before/ after	Extended or Maximum Kumbhāka	Duration of Practice	Number of Days Practiced	Variations on Practice (e.g. Use of Moving Practices in Combination with Nostril Techniques)
Write your reflection on this type of prāṇāyāma practice here:						
Write your reflection on this type of prāṇāyāma practice here:						

Type of Prāṇāyāma Technique	CP before/ after	HR before/ after	Extended or Maximum Kumbhāka	Duration of Practice	Number of Days Practiced	Variations on Practice (e.g. Use of Moving Practices in Combination with Nostril Techniques)
Write your reflection on this type of prāṇāyāma practice here:						
Write your reflection on this type of prāṇāyāma practice here:						

Type of Prāṇāyāma Technique	CP before/ after	HR before/ after	Extended or Maximum Kumbhāka	Duration of Practice	Number of Days Practiced	Variations on Practice (e.g. Use of Moving Practices in Combination with Nostril Techniques)
Write your reflection on this type of prāṇāyāma practice here:						
Write your reflection on this type of prāṇāyāma practice here:						

Type of Prāṇāyāma Technique	CP before/ after	HR before/ after	Extended or Maximum Kumbhāka	Duration of Practice	Number of Days Practiced	Variations on Practice (e.g. Use of Moving Practices in Combination with Nostril Techniques)
Write your reflection on this type of prāṇāyāma practice here:						
Write your reflection on this type of prāṇāyāma practice here:						

Type of Prāṇāyāma Technique	CP before/ after	HR before/ after	Extended or Maximum Kumbhāka	Duration of Practice	Number of Days Practiced	Variations on Practice (e.g. Use of Moving Practices in Combination with Nostril Techniques)
Write your reflection on this type of prāṇāyāma practice here:						
Write your reflection on this type of prāṇāyāma practice here:						

Type of Prāṇāyāma Technique	CP before/ after	HR before/ after	Extended or Maximum Kumbhāka	Duration of Practice	Number of Days Practiced	Variations on Practice (e.g. Use of Moving Practices in Combination with Nostril Techniques)
Write your reflection on this type of prāṇāyāma practice here:						
Write your reflection on this type of prāṇāyāma practice here:						

Type of Prāṇāyāma Technique	CP before/ after	HR before/ after	Extended or Maximum Kumbhāka	Duration of Practice	Number of Days Practiced	Variations on Practice (e.g. Use of Moving Practices in Combination with Nostril Techniques)
Write your reflection on this type of prāṇāyāma practice here:						
Write your reflection on this type of prāṇāyāma practice here:						

Type of Prāṇāyāma Technique	CP before/ after	HR before/ after	Extended or Maximum Kumbhāka	Duration of Practice	Number of Days Practiced	Variations on Practice (e.g. Use of Moving Practices in Combination with Nostril Techniques)
Write your reflection on this type of prāṇāyāma practice here:						
Write your reflection on this type of prāṇāyāma practice here:						

Type of Prāṇāyāma Technique	CP before/ after	HR before/ after	Extended or Maximum Kumbhāka	Duration of Practice	Number of Days Practiced	Variations on Practice (e.g. Use of Moving Practices in Combination with Nostril Techniques)
Write your reflection on this type of prāṇāyāma practice here:						
Write your reflection on this type of prāṇāyāma practice here:						

Glossary

abhinevesha (*ah-bhee-na-vaysh-ah*) Fear, ultimately the fear of death.

agni (*ahg-nee*) Digestive fire.

agni sara (*ahg-nee sar-ah*) A traditional practice that is used to heat the abdominal cavity. It requires a repetitive pumping action of the abdominal muscles and diaphragm and is done on breath suspension.

ahaṃkāra (*ah-hahm-kar-ah*) The ego or "I maker." According to Vedic philosophy, this is the part of the mind that allows us to think of ourselves as separate and say, "I am afraid," or "That's mine."

ahimsā (*ah-him-sah*) Non-violence, cultivation of compassion and empathy for others.

ajña (*ahj-nah*) The sixth chakra, known as the command wheel and located in the third-eye region.

alabdhabhūmikatva (*ah-lob-da-boom-ee-cot-vah*) Failing to meet the goals of practice.

ālasaya (*aw-la-sigh-ya*) Sloth, laziness.

ama (*ah-ma*) Waste.

amrit (*ahm-rit*) The divine nectar that flows from the sinuses down into the back of the throat.

anahata (*ahn-aw-hah-tah*) The fourth chakra, known as the wheel of unstruck sound and often referred to as the lotus of the heart. Located in heart region.

ānandamaya (*aw-nahn-dah-mai-yah*) The fifth maya and most subtle dimension of our being, composed of bliss or joy.

anavasthitatvāni (*ah-nah-vahs-teet-aht-vawn-ee*) Inability to maintain inner stability once attained.

annamaya (*ahn-nah-mai-ya*) The first maya or dimension of prakṛti, which encompasses the "food body" or structural body.

antarāyāh (*ahn-tar-ai-yah*) The obstacles that interfere with practice and progress.

anuloma ujjayi (*ahn-u-low-mah oo-jai-yee*) A form of prāṇāyāma practice that involves alternate nostril exhale and ujjayi inhale.

apāna (*ah-pawn-ah*) The aspect of prāṇa responsible for eliminating waste products from the body.

apānavayu (*ah-pawn-ah vai-yoo*) The wind of prāṇa that governs downward flow, elimination.

aparigrahā (*ah-par-i-grah-haw*) Living simply with what we need rather than hoarding what we want.

āsana (*aw-sah-nah*) Seat or posture. The ability to sit with stability and ease in order to practice prāṇāyāma and meditation. Commonly refers to the postures of hatha yoga practice.

asmitā (*ah-smee-taw*) I-am-ness. The awareness of oneself as a distinct being.

asteya (*ah-stay-ah*) Integrity in action; not taking what has not been offered to one.

avidya (*ah-vid-yah*) Ignorance.

avirati (*ah-vir-ah-tee*) Sensuality, craving.

bandhas (*bahn-dahs*) Muscular locks.

bastrika (*bah-streek-ah*) A cleansing breath practice commonly called Bellow's Breath.

bhāvana (*baw-vah-nah*) Cultivation, what we dwell upon, our intention.

bhrānti darśana (*brawn-tee dar-sha-nah*) False or distorted perception.

bija (*bee-jah*) Seed.

brahmacharya (*bra-mah-char-yah*) Conservation of energy; abstaining from actions that deplete us or infringe on others.

brahmari (*brah-mar-ee*) The Bee Breath or humming.

buddhi (*bood-deeh*) According to Vedic philosophy, this is the discriminating aspect of the mind that allows for higher, rational thinking.

chakras (*chah-krahs*) The energy centers.

chandra bhedana (*cha-n-drah bayd-ah-nah*) A prāṇāyāma practice that involves breathing in and out of the left nostril.

citta (*chi [short "i"] -ta*) Mind.

dīrgha (*deer-gah*) Long (refers to the ability to sustain the space between breaths).

dośa (*doe-shah*) Ayurvedic term referring to the three bodily humors (or elemental constitutions) of vata (air + space), pitta (fire + water), and kapha (earth + water).

duḥkha (*dooh-khah*) Suffering or stuckness.

dveṣa (*d-vesh-ah*) Aversion.

guṇas (*goo-nahs*) The three energetic qualities of prakṛti or nature (lucidity, action, and inertia).

hṛdaya (*h-rid-ayah*) Heart.

iḍā nādi (*ee-dah nah-dee*) According to esoteric anatomy, this is one of the three major channels of energy running through the body. It is connected to the left nostril and is associated with cooling, quieting, feminine, and receptive energies.

īśvarapraṇidhāna (*esh-va-ra-pra-nee-dha-na*) Dedication to God.

jālandhara bandha (*jawl-ahn-dah-rah bahn-dah*) A hatha yoga technique—the action of "locking the throat" in order to contain energy.

Jiva Mūdra (*jee-vah moo-drah*) The position of the flat of the tongue pressing firmly into the upper palate.

kapālabhāti (*kah-pall-ah-bah-tee*) A cleansing breath practice commonly called the Skull Shining Breath.

kapha (*kah-pha*) One of the three ayurvedic dośas (bodily humors or elemental constitutions), kapha is made of earth and water, and has the qualities of heavy, cold, oily, and sweet.

Kechari Mūdra (*kay-char-ee moo-drah*) You could think of this as a "tongue lift," as it requires stretching the tongue up into the cavity of the soft palate.

kleśas (*kley-shas*) Afflictions or impediments. The Yoga Sūtras list five of them: ignorance, ego, attachment, aversion, and clinging to life.

krama (*krah-mah*) A stepped, segmented, or staged action.

kriya yoga (*kree-yah yo-ga*) The yoga of action.

kumbhāka (*koom-baw-kah*) Retention or suspension of breath. Used synonymously with prāṇāyāma in the Vedic texts.

kundalini rising (*koon-da-lee-nee rising*) A common phrase used in many yoga traditions to indicate the state of enlightenment which occurs when prāṇa from iḍā and piṅgalā culminate in the suṣumnā nādi and the energy moves up through the chakra centers to the sahāsrara, the crown center.

maṇipūra (*mah-nee-poor-ah*) The third chakra, known as the wheel of the jeweled city and located in the navel region.

manomaya (*mah-no-mai-yah*) The mental, sensory sheath of our being.

mantra (*mahn-trah*) Mental recitation that takes us out of our ordinary thought process, and connects us to something less fear-driven, like Light, Love, Peace, or God.

mūlabandha (*moo-lah-bahn-dah*) A hatha yoga technique referring to the action of "locking the root" in order to contain energy.

mūladhāra (*moo-lah-dah-rah*) The first chakra. Considered the root center and located at the base of the spine, near the coccyx.

nādi (*nah-dee*) Literally means "a river, channel, passageway, or pulse."

nādi shodhāna (*nah-dee show-dah-nah*) A form of prāṇāyāma practice that involves alternate nostril inhale and exhale.

panchamaya (*pawn-cha-maiy-a*) The dimensions of prakṛti; also known as the koshas in some lineages.

panchavāyus (*pawn-cha-vai-yoos*) The five winds that move energy through us.

Patañjali (*pah-tawn-jah-lee*) The ancient sage credited with writing the Yoga Sūtras.

piṅgalā (*pin-ga-law*) Sūrya/sun, heating, SNS, stimulating.

pitta (*pit-tah*) One of the three ayurvedic dośas (bodily humors or elemental constitutions), pitta is made of fire and water, and has the qualities of hot, pungent, and liquid.

prakṛti (*pra-kri-tee*) Nature.

pramāda (*pra-maw-da*) Carelessness, negligence, lack of interest.

prāṇ (*prawn*) Synonymous with prāna, the principal life air or life-force.

prāṇa (*prawn-ah*) Principal life air or life-force.

prāṇa shakti (*prawn-ah shahk-tee*) Great prāṇic energy.

prāṇa vidya (*prawn-ah vid-yah*) Knowledge of prāṇa.

prāṇamaya (*prawn-ah-maiy-a*) The vital, energetic sheath of our being.

prāṇavayu (*prawn-ah-vai-yoo*) The wind of prāṇa that governs inward flow, ingestion.

prāṇāyāma (*prawn-aw-yaw-mah*) The practice of breath control.

pratikriya (*prah-tee-kree-ya*) Opposite action.

pratiloma ujjayi (*prah-tee-lo-mah oo-jai-yee*) A complex form of prāṇāyāma practice that combines anuloma and viloma ujjayi.

pratyāhāra (*prah-tee-ah-har-ah*) Sense withdrawal.

prithivī (*prih-tih-vee*) Earth.

puruṣa (*pu-roo-sha*) The opposite of nature (prakṛti). Self, soul, pure awareness, unbound consciousness.

raga (*ra-ga [hard "g"]*) Interpreted in most texts as attachment, raga speaks to our tendency to become attached to the experiences that we consider pleasant or pleasurable.

rajas (*rah-jahs*) Movement.

sādhanā (*sah-dah-nah*) Practice.

sahāsrara (*sah-haws-ra-rah*) The seventh chakra, known as the thousand-spoked wheel or the thousand-petaled lotus and located in the crown of the head.

samāna/samānavayu (*sah-maw-nah/sah-maw-nah-vai-yoo*) The wind of prāṇa responsible for digestion.

Sāṁkhya (*san-khi-ya*) One of six classical Indian philosophies designed to explain the nature of reality.

samśāya (*sum-shy-ah*) Indecision, doubt, skepticism.

saṃskāra (*sum-scar-ah*) Mental imprints or impressions created in the subconscious through every experience or thought we have.

Sarvāṅgāsana (*sar-vahn-gah-sahnah*) Shoulderstand—used as a counter pose for Śīrṣāsana.

sattva (*saht-vah*) Light, balance. The energetic quality of clarity and illumination.

satya (*saht-yah*) Truthful communication; refraining from gossip, speaking with ahimsa.

Shalambhāsana (*sha-lahm-bhaw-sah-nah*) Locust pose.

shat-karmas (*shaht-kar-mahs*) Cleansing practices, used to reduce phlegm and congestion, and to aid digestion and elimination.

shītali (*shee-ta-lee*) The intake through the tongue, which is also funneled and highly controlled.

shītkari (*sheet-kar-ee*) An adaptation of shītali practice for those who are unable to perform the tongue curl.

Śīrṣāsana (*sheer-sha-sahnah*) Headstand.

styāna (*stee-yawn-ah*) Inefficiency, mental dullness.

sūkṣma (*sook-shmah*) Subtle.

sūrya bhedana (*sooryah bayd-ah-nah*) A prāṇāyāma practice that involves breathing in and out of the right nostril.

suṣumnā (*suh-shum-naw*) According to esoteric anatomy, this is the major channel of energy running from the base of the spine to the crown of the head.

sūtra (*soo-trah*) Literally means "thread," and refers to a style of writing employed in the major source books of Indian philosophy.

svādhiṣṭhāna (*s-vah-dih-staw-nah*) The second chakra, known as the "own-base center" and located in the genital region.

svādhyāya (*s-vah-dhee-yaw-yah*) Translates as "self-reflection."

Tadāsana (*tah-daw-sah-nah*) Mountain pose.

tamas (*tah-mahs*) The quality of inertia, encompassing lethargy, dullness, and the state of deep sleep.

tapas (*tah-pahs*) Cultivation of willpower over the pull of the senses through practice.

udāna (*oo-dawn-ah*) The aspect of prāṇa responsible for upward movements in the body.

uḍḍiyāna bandha (*ood-dee-yaw-nah bahn-dah*) A hatha yoga technique referring to the action of "locking the abdominals" in order to contain energy.

Utkatāsana (*oot-kah-tah-sah-nah*) Chair pose.

vata (*vah-tah*) One of the three ayurvedic dośas (bodily humors or elemental constitutions), vata is made of air and space, and has the qualities of dryness, coldness, and mobility.

vāyus (*vai-yoos*) Forces of air, wind.

vidya (*vid-yah*) Knowledge, wisdom.

vijñānamaya (*vig-nah-na-mai-yah*) The fourth maya or dimension of prakṛti, which encompasses our intuition, innate understanding, and wisdom.

viloma ujjayi (*vi-lo-mah oo-jai-yee*) A form of prāṇāyāma practice that involves alternate nostril inhale and ujjayi exhale.

vīrya (*veer-yah*) Vitality and energy.

viśhuddhi (*vi-shood-dhee*) The fifth chakra, known as the pure wheel or wheel of purity and located in the throat region.

vṛttis (*v-rit-tees*) Literally means whirl, referring to the habitual patterns of thought that swirl through the mind.

vyādhi (*vi-yah-dee*) Disease, illness, sickness.

vyāna (*vee-yawn-ah*) The aspect of prāṇa responsible for circulation and assimilation.

yama (*yah-mah*) The first limb of yoga, referring to the five outward disciplines.

Endnotes

Chapter 3

1 At sea level and with good air quality, oxygen constitutes only 21 percent of the air we breathe. The major component of our atmosphere is nitrogen, at 78 percent.

2 Blood levels of O_2 have to drop significantly, by about 30–50 percent, before our brain will increase our ventilatory response (call to breathe).

3 The CP or Comfortable/Control Pause was conceived by the late Dr. Konstantin Buteyko, a Russian physician. In the 1950s Dr. Buteyko developed the Buteyko Breathing Method to address respiratory ailments such as chronic obstructive pulmonary disease (COPD), asthma, and various cardiovascular conditions. To learn more about the Buteyko Method, please contact the Buteyko Breathing Educators Association at https://buteykoeducators.org.

Chapter 4

1 Jones, M., Harvey, A., Marston, L. & O'Connell, N.E. (2013) Breathing exercises for dysfunctional breathing/hyperventilation syndrome in adults. *Cochrane Database of Systematic Reviews 31* (5), CD009041.

2 Felcar, J., Bueno, I., Massan, A., Torezan, R. & Cardoso, J. (2010) Prevalence of mouth breathing in children from an elementary school. *Cien Saude Colet 15* (2), 437–444.

Abreu, R.R., Rocha, R.L., Lamounier, J.A. & Guerra, A.F. (2008) Prevalence of mouth breathing among children. *Jornal de Pediatria 84* (5), 467–470.

De Menezes, V.A., Leal, R.B., Pessoac, R.S. & Pontes, R.M. (2006) Prevalence and factors related to mouth breathing in school children at the Santo Amaro project-Recife. *Brazilian Journal of Otorhinolaryngology 72* (3), 394–398.

3 Johnson, B.D., Scanlon, P.D. & Beck, K.C. (1995) Regulation of ventilatory capacity during exercise in asthmatics. *Journal of Applied Physiology 79* (3), 892–901.

Bowler, S.D., Green, A. & Mitchell, C.A. (1998) Buteyko breathing techniques in asthma: A blinded randomised controlled trial. *Medical Journal of Australia 169,* 575–578.

Mcnicholas, W.T., Coffey, M. & Boyle, T. (1993) Effects of nasal airflow on breathing during sleep in normal humans. *American Review of Respiratory Disease 147* (3), 620–623.

Jordan, A.S., McEvoy, R.D., Edwards, J.K., Schory, K. *et al.* (2004) The influence of gender and upper airway resistance on the ventilatory response to arousal in obstructive sleep apnoea in humans. *Journal of Physiology 558* (Pt 3), 993–1004.

Radwan, L., Maszczyk, Z., Koziorowski, A., Koziej, M. *et al.* (1995) Control of breathing in obstructive sleep apnea and in patients with the overlap syndrome. *European Respiratory Journal 8* (4), 542–545.

4 Timmons, B.H. & Ley, R. (1994) *Behavioral and Psychological Approaches to Breathing Disorders.* New York, NY: Plenum Press. p. 4.

5 Lum, L.C. (1987) Hyperventilation syndromes in medicine and psychiatry: A review. *Journal of the Royal Society of Medicine 80* (4), 229–231.

Santiago, T.V. & Edelman, N.H. (1986) Brain Blood Flow and Control of Breathing. In A.P. Fishman (ed.) *Handbook of Physiology, vol. 3, part 1, The Respiratory System.* Bethesda, MA: American Physiological Society. pp. 163–179.

6 Saraswati, N. (2010) *Prāṇa and Prāṇāyāma.* Munger, Bihar: Yoga Publication Trust. pp. 190–195.

Chapter 5

1 Courtney, R. (1997) Optimise your breathing and gain control of your health using the Buteyko breathing method. *Wellbeing Magazine 68* (June). https://buteykoclinic.com/buteyko-method

2 Felcar, J., Bueno, I., Massan, A., Torezan, R. & Cardoso, J. (2010) Prevalence of mouth breathing in children from an elementary school. *Cien Saude Colet 15* (2), 437–444.

Jefferson Y. (2010) Mouth breathing: Adverse effects on facial growth, health, academics, and behavior. *General Dentistry 58*, 18–25.

Chapter 6

1 Lindgren, H. (2011) Diaphragm function for core stability. Accessed on November 12, 2019 at http://hanslindgren.com/articles/diaphragm-function-for-core-stability

Courtney, R. (2017) Breathing training for dysfunctional breathing in asthma: Taking a multidimensional approach. *ERJ Open Research 3*. doi.org/10.1183/23120541.00065-2017.

2 Lindgren, H. (2011) Diaphragm function for core stability. Accessed on November 12, 2019 at http://hanslindgren.com/articles/diaphragm-function-for-core-stability

Courtney, R. (2017) Breathing training for dysfunctional breathing in asthma: Taking a multidimensional approach. *ERJ Open Research 3*. doi.org/10.1183/23120541.00065-2017.

Nagarwala, R., Dhotre, P. & Gelani, I. (2011) Correlation between core strength and breath holding time in normal young adults. *Journal of Orthopedics and Rehabilitation 1* (1), 75–78.

3 My utilization of undulation is derived from Anita Boser's book *Undulation: Relieve Stiffness and Feel Young* (Issaquah, WA: Vital Self). Anita is a Board Certified Structural Integrator (BCSI) and yoga teacher. I have taken what I have learned from studying with Anita and created my own undulation movements, which are now a routine part of my yoga therapy work.

Chapter 7

1 Myers, T.W. (2014) *Anatomy Trains: Myofascial Meridians for Manual and Movement Therapists*. Edinburgh: Churchill Livingstone/Elsevier.

2 I intentionally use fractional percentages to ward off the tendency for students to get caught up in thinking there is an exact 30 percent or 65 percent that is just "right." This process cultivates awareness much like an undulation. I urge you to not get attached to a precise percentage, but rather to experience that middle ground between all or nothing. Explore the infinite possibilities between 0 and 100 percent, maintaining a playful attitude. This will help to keep your parasympathetic relaxation response engaged.

Chapter 8

1 Le Doux, J. (1996) *The Emotional Brain: The Mysterious Underpinnings of Emotional Life*. New York, NY: Simon & Schuster. p. 161.

2 Van der Kolk, B. (2015) *The Body Keeps the Score: Brain, Mind, and Body in the Healing of Trauma*. New York, NY: Penguin Books. p. 62.

3 Le Doux, J. (1996) *The Emotional Brain. The Mysterious Underpinnings of Emotional Life*. New York, NY: Simon & Schuster.

Davidson, R.J. & Lutz, A. (2008) Buddha's brain: Neuroplasticity and meditation. *IEEE Signal Processing Magazine 25* (1), 176–174.

4 *Vagal brake* is a term coined by Steven Porges to describe an intentional shift from low-road to high-road functioning. Porges, S.W. (2007) The polyvagal perspective. *Biological Psychology 74* (2), 116–143.

Chapter 9

1 Le Page, J. & Le Page, L. (2014) *Mudras for Healing and Transformation*. Sebastopol, CA: Integrative Yoga Therapy.

Arora, I. (2015) *Mudra: The Sacred Secret*. Bedford, MA: Yogsadhna LLC.

2 The use of ujjayi involves the contraction of the glottis, which assists diaphragmatic recruitment. While it has commonly been called the "Darth Vadar breath" and many yoga teachers encourage an audible sound while working with ujjayi, according to the yoga texts it is intended to be subtle and quiet. Limit yourself to a light contraction of the glottis, which will increase your control of the breath, and the sensation of the breath as it flows through the back of the throat, without creating any outward sound.

Chapter 10

1 Dass, H. & Diffenbaugh, D. (1999) *The Yoga Sūtras of Patañjali: A Study Guide for Book II: Samādhi Pāda.* Santa Cruz, CA: Sri Rama Publishing. Sūtra 2:52–2.53, p. 191.

2 McKeown, P. (2015) *The Oxygen Advantage: The Simple, Scientifically Proven Breathing Techniques for a Healthier, Slimmer, Faster, and Fitter You.* New York, NY: William Morrow.

3 Verges, S., Chacaroun, S., Godin-Ribuot, D. & Baillieul, S. (2015) Hypoxic conditioning as a new therapeutic modality. *Frontiers in Pediatrics 3,* 58. doi: 10.3389/fped.2015.00058.

Basovich, S.N. (2010) The role of hypoxia in mental development and in the treatment of mental disorders: A review. *Bioscience Trends 4,* 288–296.

Bailey, D.P., Smith, L.R., Chrismas, B.C., Taylor, L. *et al.* (2015) Appetite and gut hormone responses to moderate-intensity continuous exercise versus high-intensity interval exercise, in normoxic and hypoxic conditions. *Appetite 89,* 237–245. doi: 10.1016/j.appet.2015.02.019.

4 University of Colorado Denver (2011) Living at high altitude reduces risk of dying from heart disease: Low oxygen may spur genes to create blood vessels. *ScienceDaily,* 26 March 2011.

5 https://buteykoclinic.com/exercise-reduced-breathing-for-children